Practice the NET!
Nursing Entrance Test Practice Test Questions

Complete Test Preparation

Victoria BC Canada

Copyright © 2011 by Brian Stocker. ALL RIGHTS RESERVED. No part of this book may be reproduced or transferred in any form or by any means, graphic, electronic, or mechanical, including photocopying, recording, web distribution, taping, or by any information storage retrieval system, without the written permission of the author.

Notice: Complete Test Preparation makes every reasonable effort to obtain from reliable sources accurate, complete, and timely information about the tests covered in this book. Nevertheless, changes can be made in the tests or the administration of the tests at any time and Complete Test Preparation makes no representation or warranty, either expressed or implied as the accuracy, timeliness, or completeness of the information contained in this book. Complete Test Preparation makes no representations or warranties of any kind, express or implied, about the completeness, accuracy, reliability, suitability or availability with respect to the information contained in this document for any purpose. Any reliance you place on such information is therefore strictly at your own risk.

The author(s) shall not be liable for any loss incurred as a consequence of the use and application, directly or indirectly, of any information presented in this work. Sold with the understanding, the author is not engaged in rendering professional services or advice. If advice or expert assistance is required, the services of a competent professional should be sought.

The company, product and service names used in this web site are for identification purposes only. All trademarks and registered trademarks are the property of their respective owners. Complete Test Preparation is not affiliated with any educational institution.

We strongly recommend that students check with exam providers for up-to-date information regarding test content.

ISBN-13: 978-1479255986
ISBN-10: 147925598X

Version 6.6 September 2016

Published by
Complete Test Preparation Inc.
Victoria BC Canada

Visit us on the web at
http://www.test-preparation.ca
Printed in the USA

About Complete Test Preparation

The Complete Test Preparation Team has been publishing high quality study materials since 2005. Millions of students have visit our websites every year, and thousands of students, teachers and parents all over the world have purchased our teaching materials, curriculum, study guides and practice tests.

Complete Test Preparation is committed to providing to providing students with the best study materials and practice tests available on the market. Members of our team combine years of teaching experience, with experienced writers and editors, all with advanced degrees (Masters or higher).

Contents

6 **Getting Started**
The NET Study Plan 7
Making a Study Schedule 9

12 **Practice Test Questions Set 1**
Answer Key 50

66 **Practice Test Questions Set 2**
Answer Key 104

117 **Conclusion**

Getting Started

CONGRATULATIONS! By deciding to take the Nursing Entrance Test (NET) Exam, you have taken the first step toward a great future! Of course, there is no point in taking this important examination unless you intend to do your very best in order to earn the highest grade you possibly can. That means getting yourself organized and discovering the best approaches, methods and strategies to master the material. Yes, that will require real effort and dedication on your part but if you are willing to focus your energy and devote the study time necessary, before you know it you will be opening that letter of acceptance to the school of your dreams.

We know that taking on a new endeavour can be a little scary, and it is easy to feel unsure of where to begin. That's where we come in. This study guide is designed to help you improve your test-taking skills, show you a few tricks of the trade and increase both your competency and confidence.

The Nursing Entrance Test Exam

The NET exam is composed of modules and not all schools use all modules. It is therefore very important that you find out what modules your school will use! That way you won't waste valuable study time learning something that isn't on your exam!

The NET has just one standard module, mathematics, and three optional modules, which are, Grammar, Punctuation and Reading Comprehension.

You don`t have to worry because these sections are included in this study guide. However, to maximize your study time, it is very important to check which modules your university offers before studying everything under the sun!

While we seek to make our guide as comprehensive as possible, it is important to note that like all entrance exams, the NET Exam might be adjusted at some future point. New material might be added, or content that is no longer relevant or applicable might be removed. It is always a good idea to give the materials you receive when you register to take the NET a careful review.

The NET Study Plan

Now that you have made the decision to take the NET, it is time to get started. Before you do another thing, you will need to figure out a plan of attack. The very best study tip is to start early! The longer the time period you devote to regular study practice, the more likely you will be to retain the material and be able to access it quickly. If you thought that 1x20 is the same as 2x10, guess what? It really is not, when it comes to study time. Reviewing material for just an hour per day over the course of 20 days is far better than studying for two hours a day for only 10 days. The more often you revisit a particular piece of information, the better you will know it. Not only will your grasp and understanding be better, but your ability to reach into your brain and quickly and efficiently pull out the tidbit you need, will be greatly enhanced as well.

The great Chinese scholar and philosopher Confucius believed that true knowledge could be defined as knowing both what you know and what you do not know. The first step in preparing for the NET Exam is to assess your strengths and weaknesses. You may already have an idea of what you know and what you do not know, but evaluating yourself using our Self- Assessment modules for each of the three areas, Math, English and Reading Comprehension, will clarify the details.

Making a Study Schedule

In order to make your study time most productive you will need to develop a study plan. The purpose of the plan is to organize all the bits of pieces of information in such a way that you will not feel overwhelmed. Rome was not built in a day, and learning everything you will need to know in order to pass the NET Exam is going to take time, too. Arranging the material you need to learn into manageable chunks is the best way to go. Each study session should make you feel as though you have succeeded in accomplishing your goal, and your goal is simply to learn what you planned to learn during that particular session. Try to organize the content in such a way that each study session builds upon previous ones. That way, you will retain the information, be better able to access it, and review the previous bits and pieces at the same time.

Self-assessment

The Best Study Tip! The very best study tip is to start early! The longer you study regularly, the more you will retain and 'learn' the material. Studying for 1 hour per day for 20 days is far better than studying for 2 hours for 10 days.

What don't you know?

The first step is to assess your strengths and weaknesses. You may already have an idea of where your weaknesses are, or you can take our Self-assessment modules for each of the areas, Math, English (Optional) and Reading Comprehension (Optional).

Exam Component	Rate from 1 to 5
Reading Comprehension	
(Optional)	
Paragraph & Passage Comprehension	
Drawing Inferences & Conclusions	
English (optional)	
Punctuation (Optional)	
English Grammar (Optional)	
Math	
Metric Conversion	
Algebra	
Fractions	
Decimals	
Percent	

Making a Study Schedule

The key to making a study plan is to divide the material you need to learn into manageable size and learn it, while at the same time reviewing the material that you already know.

Using the table above, any scores of 3 or below, you need to spend time learning, going over and practicing this subject area. A score of 4 means you need to review the material, but you don't have to spend time re-learning. A score of 5 and you are OK with just an occasional review before the exam.

A score of 0 or 1 means you really need to work on this area and should allocate the most time and the highest priority. Some students prefer a 5-day plan and others a 10-day plan. It also depends on how much time you have until the exam.

Here is an example of a 5-day plan based on an example from the table above:

Fractions: 1 Study 1 hour everyday – review on last day
Punctuation: 3 Study 1 hour for 2 days then ½ hour a day, then review
Percent: 4 Review every second day
Word Problems: 2 Study 1 hour on the first day – then ½ hour everyday
Reading Comprehension: 5 Review for ½ hour every other day
Algebra: 5 Review for ½ hour every other day
Grammar: 5 very confident – review a few times.

Using this example, Algebra and Grammar are good and only need occasional review. Punctuation is also good and needs 'some' review. Decimals need a bit of work, Word Problems need a lot of work and Fractions are very weak and need the majority of time. Based on this, here is a sample study plan:

Day	Subject	Time
Monday		
Study	Fractions	1 hour
Study	Word Problems	1 hour
	½ **hour break**	
Study	Punctuation	1 hour
Review	Grammar	½ hour
Tuesday		
Study	Fractions	1 hour
Study	Word Problems	½ hour
	½ **hour break**	
Study	Decimals	½ hour
Review	Percent	½ hour
Review	Grammar	½ hour
Wednesday		
Study	Fractions	1 hour
Study	Word Problems	½ hour
	½ **hour break**	
Study	Punctuation	½ hour

Review	Grammar	½ hour
Thursday		
Study	Fractions	½ hour
Study	Word Problems	½ hour
Review	Punctuation	½ hour
	½ hour break	
Review	Grammar	½ hour
Review	Percent	½ hour
Friday		
Review	Fractions	½ hour
Review	Word Problems	½ hour
Review	Punctuation	½ hour
	½ hour break	
Review	Percent	½ hour
Review	Grammar	½ hour

Practice Test Questions Set 1

THE PRACTICE TEST PORTION PRESENTS QUESTIONS THAT ARE REPRESENTATIVE OF THE TYPE OF QUESTION YOU SHOULD EXPECT TO FIND ON THE NET. However, they are not intended to match exactly what is on the NET.

For the best results, take this Practice Test as if it were the real exam. Set aside time when you will not be disturbed, and a location that is quiet and free of distractions. Read the instructions carefully, read each question carefully, and answer to the best of your ability.

Use the bubble answer sheets provided. When you have completed the Practice Test, check your answer against the Answer Key and read the explanation provided.

NOTE: The Reading Comprehension, English and Punctuation sections are optional. Check with your school for exam details.

Reading Comprehension Answer Sheet

1. Ⓐ Ⓑ Ⓒ Ⓓ   11. Ⓐ Ⓑ Ⓒ Ⓓ   21. Ⓐ Ⓑ Ⓒ Ⓓ

2. Ⓐ Ⓑ Ⓒ Ⓓ   12. Ⓐ Ⓑ Ⓒ Ⓓ   22. Ⓐ Ⓑ Ⓒ Ⓓ

3. Ⓐ Ⓑ Ⓒ Ⓓ   13. Ⓐ Ⓑ Ⓒ Ⓓ   23. Ⓐ Ⓑ Ⓒ Ⓓ

4. Ⓐ Ⓑ Ⓒ Ⓓ   14. Ⓐ Ⓑ Ⓒ Ⓓ   24. Ⓐ Ⓑ Ⓒ Ⓓ

5. Ⓐ Ⓑ Ⓒ Ⓓ   15. Ⓐ Ⓑ Ⓒ Ⓓ   25. Ⓐ Ⓑ Ⓒ Ⓓ

6. Ⓐ Ⓑ Ⓒ Ⓓ   16. Ⓐ Ⓑ Ⓒ Ⓓ   26. Ⓐ Ⓑ Ⓒ Ⓓ

7. Ⓐ Ⓑ Ⓒ Ⓓ   17. Ⓐ Ⓑ Ⓒ Ⓓ   27. Ⓐ Ⓑ Ⓒ Ⓓ

8. Ⓐ Ⓑ Ⓒ Ⓓ   18. Ⓐ Ⓑ Ⓒ Ⓓ   28. Ⓐ Ⓑ Ⓒ Ⓓ

9. Ⓐ Ⓑ Ⓒ Ⓓ   19. Ⓐ Ⓑ Ⓒ Ⓓ   29. Ⓐ Ⓑ Ⓒ Ⓓ

10. Ⓐ Ⓑ Ⓒ Ⓓ   20. Ⓐ Ⓑ Ⓒ Ⓓ   30. Ⓐ Ⓑ Ⓒ Ⓓ

Math Answer Sheet

1. Ⓐ Ⓑ Ⓒ Ⓓ   21. Ⓐ Ⓑ Ⓒ Ⓓ
2. Ⓐ Ⓑ Ⓒ Ⓓ   22. Ⓐ Ⓑ Ⓒ Ⓓ
3. Ⓐ Ⓑ Ⓒ Ⓓ   23. Ⓐ Ⓑ Ⓒ Ⓓ
4. Ⓐ Ⓑ Ⓒ Ⓓ   24. Ⓐ Ⓑ Ⓒ Ⓓ
5. Ⓐ Ⓑ Ⓒ Ⓓ   25. Ⓐ Ⓑ Ⓒ Ⓓ
6. Ⓐ Ⓑ Ⓒ Ⓓ   26. Ⓐ Ⓑ Ⓒ Ⓓ
7. Ⓐ Ⓑ Ⓒ Ⓓ   27. Ⓐ Ⓑ Ⓒ Ⓓ
8. Ⓐ Ⓑ Ⓒ Ⓓ   28. Ⓐ Ⓑ Ⓒ Ⓓ
9. Ⓐ Ⓑ Ⓒ Ⓓ   29. Ⓐ Ⓑ Ⓒ Ⓓ
10. Ⓐ Ⓑ Ⓒ Ⓓ   30. Ⓐ Ⓑ Ⓒ Ⓓ
11. Ⓐ Ⓑ Ⓒ Ⓓ   31. Ⓐ Ⓑ Ⓒ Ⓓ
12. Ⓐ Ⓑ Ⓒ Ⓓ   32. Ⓐ Ⓑ Ⓒ Ⓓ
13. Ⓐ Ⓑ Ⓒ Ⓓ   33. Ⓐ Ⓑ Ⓒ Ⓓ
14. Ⓐ Ⓑ Ⓒ Ⓓ   34. Ⓐ Ⓑ Ⓒ Ⓓ
15. Ⓐ Ⓑ Ⓒ Ⓓ   35. Ⓐ Ⓑ Ⓒ Ⓓ
16. Ⓐ Ⓑ Ⓒ Ⓓ   36. Ⓐ Ⓑ Ⓒ Ⓓ
17. Ⓐ Ⓑ Ⓒ Ⓓ   37. Ⓐ Ⓑ Ⓒ Ⓓ
18. Ⓐ Ⓑ Ⓒ Ⓓ   38. Ⓐ Ⓑ Ⓒ Ⓓ
19. Ⓐ Ⓑ Ⓒ Ⓓ   39. Ⓐ Ⓑ Ⓒ Ⓓ
20. Ⓐ Ⓑ Ⓒ Ⓓ   40. Ⓐ Ⓑ Ⓒ Ⓓ

English Answer Sheet

1. Ⓐ Ⓑ Ⓒ Ⓓ   21. Ⓐ Ⓑ Ⓒ Ⓓ
2. Ⓐ Ⓑ Ⓒ Ⓓ   22. Ⓐ Ⓑ Ⓒ Ⓓ
3. Ⓐ Ⓑ Ⓒ Ⓓ   23. Ⓐ Ⓑ Ⓒ Ⓓ
4. Ⓐ Ⓑ Ⓒ Ⓓ   24. Ⓐ Ⓑ Ⓒ Ⓓ
5. Ⓐ Ⓑ Ⓒ Ⓓ   25. Ⓐ Ⓑ Ⓒ Ⓓ
6. Ⓐ Ⓑ Ⓒ Ⓓ   26. Ⓐ Ⓑ Ⓒ Ⓓ
7. Ⓐ Ⓑ Ⓒ Ⓓ   27. Ⓐ Ⓑ Ⓒ Ⓓ
8. Ⓐ Ⓑ Ⓒ Ⓓ   28. Ⓐ Ⓑ Ⓒ Ⓓ
9. Ⓐ Ⓑ Ⓒ Ⓓ   29. Ⓐ Ⓑ Ⓒ Ⓓ
10. Ⓐ Ⓑ Ⓒ Ⓓ   30. Ⓐ Ⓑ Ⓒ Ⓓ
11. Ⓐ Ⓑ Ⓒ Ⓓ   31. Ⓐ Ⓑ Ⓒ Ⓓ
12. Ⓐ Ⓑ Ⓒ Ⓓ   32. Ⓐ Ⓑ Ⓒ Ⓓ
13. Ⓐ Ⓑ Ⓒ Ⓓ   33. Ⓐ Ⓑ Ⓒ Ⓓ
14. Ⓐ Ⓑ Ⓒ Ⓓ   34. Ⓐ Ⓑ Ⓒ Ⓓ
15. Ⓐ Ⓑ Ⓒ Ⓓ   35. Ⓐ Ⓑ Ⓒ Ⓓ
16. Ⓐ Ⓑ Ⓒ Ⓓ   36. Ⓐ Ⓑ Ⓒ Ⓓ
17. Ⓐ Ⓑ Ⓒ Ⓓ   37. Ⓐ Ⓑ Ⓒ Ⓓ
18. Ⓐ Ⓑ Ⓒ Ⓓ   38. Ⓐ Ⓑ Ⓒ Ⓓ
19. Ⓐ Ⓑ Ⓒ Ⓓ   39. Ⓐ Ⓑ Ⓒ Ⓓ
20. Ⓐ Ⓑ Ⓒ Ⓓ   40. Ⓐ Ⓑ Ⓒ Ⓓ

Section I - Reading Comprehension.

Directions: The following questions are based on a number of reading passages. Each passage is followed by a series of questions. Read each passage carefully, and then answer the questions based on it. You may reread the passage as often as you wish. When you have finished answering the questions based on one passage, go right on to the next passage. Choose the best answer based on the information given and implied.

Questions 1 – 4 refer to the following passage.

Passage 1 - Infectious Disease

An infectious disease is a clinically evident illness resulting from the presence of pathogenic agents, such as viruses, bacteria, fungi, protozoa, multi cellular parasites, and unusual proteins known as prions. Infectious pathologies are also called communicable diseases or transmissible diseases, due to their potential of transmission from one person or species to another by a replicating agent (as opposed to a toxin).

Transmission of an infectious disease can occur in many different ways. Physical contact, liquids, food, body fluids, contaminated objects, and airborne inhalation can all transmit infecting agents.

Transmissible diseases that occur through contact with an ill person, or objects touched by them, are especially infective, and are sometimes called contagious diseases. Communicable diseases that require a more specialized route of infection, such as through blood or needle transmission, or sexual transmission, are usually not regarded as contagious.

The term infectivity describes the ability of an organism to enter, survive and multiply in the host, while the infectiousness of a disease shows the comparative ease with which the disease is transmitted. An infection however, is not synonymous with an infectious disease, as an infection may not cause important clinical symptoms. [4]

1. What can we infer from the first paragraph in this passage?

    a. Sickness from a toxin can be easily transmitted from one person to another.

    b. Sickness from an infectious disease can be easily transmitted from one person to another.

    c. Few sicknesses are transmitted from one person to another.

    d. Infectious diseases are easily treated.

2. What are two other names for infections' pathologies?

    a. Communicable diseases or transmissible diseases

    b. Communicable diseases or terminal diseases

    c. Transmissible diseases or preventable diseases

    d. Communicative diseases or unstable diseases

3. What does infectivity describe?

    a. The inability of an organism to multiply in the host

    b. The inability of an organism to reproduce

    c. The ability of an organism to enter, survive and multiply in the host

    d. The ability of an organism to reproduce in the host

4. How do we know an infection is not synonymous with an infectious disease?

    a. Because an infectious disease destroys infections with enough time.

    b. Because an infection may not cause important clinical symptoms or impair host function.

    c. We do not. The two are synonymous.

    d. Because an infection is too fatal to be an infectious disease.

Questions 5 – 8 refer to the following passage.

Passage 2 - Viruses

A virus (from the Latin virus meaning toxin or poison) is a small infectious agent that can replicate only inside the living cells of other organisms. Most viruses are too small to be seen directly with a microscope. Viruses infect all types of organisms, from animals and plants to bacteria and single-celled organisms.

Unlike prions and viroids, viruses consist of two or three parts: all viruses have genes made from either DNA or RNA, all have a protein coat that protects these genes, and some have an envelope of fat that surrounds them when they are outside a cell. (Viroids do not have a protein coat and prions contain no RNA or DNA.) Viruses vary from simple to very complex structures. Most viruses are about one hundred times smaller than an average bacterium. The origins of viruses in the evolutionary history of life are unclear: some may have evolved from plasmids—pieces of DNA that can move between cells—while others may have evolved from bacteria.

Viruses spread in many ways; plant viruses are often transmitted from plant to plant by insects that feed on sap, such as aphids, while animal viruses can be carried by blood-sucking insects. These disease-bearing organisms are known as vectors. Influenza viruses are spread by coughing and sneezing. HIV is one of several viruses transmitted through sexual contact and by exposure to infected blood. Viruses can infect only a limited range of host cells called the "host range". This can be broad as when a virus is capable of infecting many species or narrow. [5]

5. What can we infer from the first paragraph in this selection?

    a. A virus is the same as bacterium

    b. A person with excellent vision can see a virus with the naked eye

    c. A virus cannot be seen with the naked eye

    d. Not all viruses are dangerous

6. What types of organisms do viruses infect?

    a. Only plants and humans

    b. Only animals and humans

    c. Only disease-prone humans

    d. All types of organisms

7. How many parts do prions and viroids consist of?

    a. Two

    b. Three

    c. Either less than two or more than three

    d. Less than two

8. What is one common virus spread by coughing and sneezing?

    a. AIDS

    b. Influenza

    c. Herpes

    d. Tuberculosis

Questions 9 – 11 refer to the following passage.

Passage 3 – Clouds

The first stage of a thunderstorm is the cumulus stage, or

developing stage. In this stage, masses of moisture are lifted upwards into the atmosphere. The trigger for this lift can be insulation heating the ground producing thermals, areas where two winds converge, forcing air upwards, or where winds blow over terrain of increasing elevation. Moisture in the air rapidly cools into liquid drops of water, which appears as cumulus clouds.

As the water vapor condenses into liquid, latent heat is released which warms the air, causing it to become less dense than the surrounding dry air. The warm air rises in an updraft through the process of convection (hence the term convective precipitation). This creates a low-pressure zone beneath the forming thunderstorm. In a typical thunderstorm, about 5×10^8 kg of water vapor is lifted, and the quantity of energy released when this condenses is about equal to the energy used by a city of 100,000 in a month. [6]

9. The cumulus stage of a thunderstorm is the

    a. The last stage of the storm

    b. The middle stage of the storm formation

    c. The beginning of the thunderstorm

    d. The period after the thunderstorm has ended

10. One of the ways the air is warmed is

    a. Air moving downwards, which will creates a high-pressure zone

    b. Air cooling and becoming less dense, causing it to rise

    c. Moisture moving downward toward the earth

    d. Heat created by water vapor condensing into liquid

11. Identify the correct sequence of events

    a. Warm air rises, water droplets condense, creating more heat, and the air rises further.

    b. Warm air rises and cools, water droplets condense, causing low pressure.

    c. Warm air rises and collects water vapor, the water vapor condenses as the air rises, which creates heat, and causes the air to rise further.

    d. None of the above.

Questions 12 – 14 refer to the following passage.

Passage 4 – US Weather Service

The United States National Weather Service classifies thunderstorms as severe when they reach a predetermined level. Usually, this means the storm is strong enough to inflict wind or hail damage. In most of the United States, a storm is considered severe if winds reach over 50 knots (58 mph or 93 km/h), hail is ¾ inch (2 cm) diameter or larger, or if meteorologists report funnel clouds or tornadoes. In the Central Region of the United States National Weather Service, the hail threshold for a severe thunderstorm is 1 inch (2.5 cm) in diameter. Though a funnel cloud or tornado indicates the presence of a severe thunderstorm, the various meteorological agencies would issue a tornado warning rather than a severe thunderstorm warning here.

Meteorologists in Canada define a severe thunderstorm as either having tornadoes, wind gusts of 90 km/h or greater, hail 2 centimeters in diameter or greater, rainfall more than 50 millimeters in 1 hour, or 75 millimeters in 3 hours.

Severe thunderstorms can develop from any type of thunderstorm. [7]

12. What is the purpose of this passage?

   a. Explaining when a thunderstorm turns into a tornado

   b. Explaining who issues storm warnings, and when these warnings should be issued

   c. Explaining when meteorologists consider a thunderstorm severe

   d. None of the above

13. It is possible to infer from this passage that

   a. Different areas and countries have different criteria for determining a severe storm

   b. Thunderstorms can include lightning and tornadoes, as well as violent winds and large hail

   c. If someone spots both a thunderstorm and a tornado, meteorological agencies will immediately issue a severe storm warning

   d. Canada has a much different alert system for severe storms, with criteria that are far less

14. What would the Central Region of the United States National Weather Service do if hail was 2.7 cm in diameter?

   a. Not issue a severe thunderstorm warning.

   b. Issue a tornado warning.

   c. Issue a severe thunderstorm warning.

   d. Sleet must also accompany the hail before the Weather Service will issue a storm warning.

Questions 15 – 18 refer to the following passage.

Passage 5 – Clouds

A cloud is a visible mass of droplets or frozen crystals floating in the atmosphere above the surface of the Earth or other planetary bodies. Another type of cloud is a mass of material in space, attracted by gravity, called interstellar clouds and nebulae. The branch of meteorology which studies clouds is called nephrology. When we are speaking of Earth clouds, water vapor is usually the condensing substance, which forms small droplets or ice crystal. These crystals are typically 0.01 mm in diameter. Dense, deep clouds reflect most light, so they appear white, at least from the top. Cloud droplets scatter light very efficiently, so the farther into a cloud light travels, the weaker it gets. This accounts for the gray or dark appearance at the base of large clouds. Thin clouds may appear to have acquired the color of their environment or background. [7]

15. What are clouds made of?

    a. Water droplets.

    b. Ice crystals.

    c. Ice crystals and water droplets.

    d. Clouds on Earth are made of ice crystals and water droplets.

16. The main idea of this passage is

    a. Condensation occurs in clouds, having an intense effect on the weather on the surface of the earth.

    b. Atmospheric gases are responsible for the gray color of clouds just before a severe storm happens.

    c. A cloud is a visible mass of droplets or frozen crystals floating in the atmosphere above the surface of the Earth or other planetary body.

    d. Clouds reflect light in varying amounts and degrees, depending on the size and concentration of the water droplets.

17. The branch of meteorology that studies clouds is called

    a. Convection

    b. Thermal meteorology

    c. Nephology

    d. Nephelometry

18. Why are clouds white on top and grey on the bottom?

    a. Because water droplets inside the cloud do not reflect light, it appears white, and the farther into the cloud the light travels, the less light is reflected making the bottom appear dark.

    b. Because water droplets outside the cloud reflect light, it appears dark, and the farther into the cloud the light travels, the more light is reflected making the bottom appear white.

    c. Because water droplets inside the cloud reflects light, making it appear white, and the farther into the cloud the light travels, the more light is reflected making the bottom appear dark.

    d. None of the above.

Questions 19 - 22 refer to the following recipe.

Chocolate Chip Cookies

3/4 cup sugar
3/4 cup packed brown sugar
1 cup butter, softened
2 large eggs, beaten
1 teaspoon vanilla extract
2 1/4 cups all-purpose flour
1 teaspoon baking soda
3/4 teaspoon salt
2 cups semisweet chocolate chips

If desired, 1 cup chopped pecans, or chopped walnuts. Preheat oven to 375 degrees.

Mix sugar, brown sugar, butter, vanilla and eggs in a large bowl. Stir in flour, baking soda, and salt. The dough will be very stiff.

Stir in chocolate chips by hand with a sturdy wooden spoon. Add the pecans, or other nuts, if desired. Stir until the chocolate chips and nuts are evenly dispersed.

Drop dough by rounded tablespoonfuls 2 inches apart onto a cookie sheet.

Bake 8 to 10 minutes or until light brown. Cookies may look underdone, but they will finish cooking after you take them out of the oven.

19. What is the correct order for adding these ingredients?

    a. Brown sugar, baking soda, chocolate chips
    b. Baking soda, brown sugar, chocolate chips
    c. Chocolate chips, baking soda, brown sugar
    d. Baking soda, chocolate chips, brown sugar

20. What does sturdy mean?

    a. Long
    b. Strong
    c. Short
    d. Wide

21. What does disperse mean?

    a. Scatter
    b. To form a ball
    c. To stir
    d. To beat

22. When can you stop stirring the nuts?

   a. When the cookies are cooked.
   b. When the nuts are evenly distributed.
   c. As soon as the nuts are added.
   d. After the chocolate chips are added.

Questions 23 – 25 refer to the following passage.

Passage 7 – Caterpillars

Butterfly larvae, or caterpillars, eat enormous quantities of leaves and spend practically all their time in search of food. Although most caterpillars are herbivorous, a few species eat other insects. Some larvae form mutual associations with ants. They communicate with ants using vibrations transmitted through the soil, as well as with chemical signals. The ants provide some degree of protection to the larvae and they in turn gather honeydew secretions. [8]

23. What do most larvae spend their time looking for?

   a. Leaves
   b. Insects
   c. Leaves and insects
   d. Honeydew secretions

24. What benefit do larvae get from association with ants?

   a. They do not receive any benefit
   b. Ants give them protection
   c. Ants give them food
   d. Ants give them honeydew secretions

25. Do ants or larvae benefit most from association?

    a. Ants benefit most.
    b. Larvae benefit most.
    c. Both benefit the same.
    d. Neither benefits.

Questions 26 – 30 refer to the following passage.

Passage 8 – Navy Seals

The United States Navy's Sea, Air and Land Teams, commonly known as Navy SEALs, are the U.S. Navy's principal special operations force, and a part of the Naval Special Warfare Command (NSWC) as well as the maritime component of the United States Special Operations Command (USSOCOM).

The unit's acronym ("SEAL") comes from their capacity to operate at sea, in the air, and on land – but it is their ability to work underwater that separates SEALs from most other military units in the world. Navy SEALs are trained and have been deployed in a wide variety of missions, including direct action and special reconnaissance operations, unconventional warfare, foreign internal defence, hostage rescue, counter-terrorism and other missions. All SEALs are members of either the United States Navy or the United States Coast Guard.

In the early morning of May 2, 2011 local time, a team of 40 CIA-led Navy SEALs completed an operation to kill Osama bin Laden in Abbottabad, Pakistan about 35 miles (56 km) from Islamabad, the country's capital. The Navy SEALs were part of the Naval Special Warfare Development Group, previously called "Team 6." President Barack Obama later confirmed the death of bin Laden. The unprecedented media coverage raised the public profile of the SEAL community, particularly the counter-terrorism specialists commonly known as SEAL Team 6. [9]

26. Are Navy SEALs part of USSOCOM?

    a. Yes

    b. No

    c. Only for special operations

    d. No, they are part of the US Navy

27. What separates Navy SEALs from other military units?

    a. Belonging to NSWC

    b. Direct action and special reconnaissance operations

    c. Working underwater

    d. Working for other military units in the world

28. What other military organizations do SEALs belong?

    a. The US Navy

    b. The Coast Guard

    c. The US Army

    d. The Navy and the Coast Guard

29. What other organization participated in the Bin Laden raid?

    a. The CIA

    b. The US Military

    c. Counter-terrorism specialists

    d. None of the above

30. What is the new name for Team 6?

    a. They were always called Team 6

    b. The counter-terrorism specialists

    c. The Naval Special Warfare Development Group

    d. None of the above

Section II – Mathematics

1. What is 1/3 of 3/4?

    a. 1/4
    b. 1/3
    c. 2/3
    d. 3/4

2. What fraction of $75 is $1500?

    a. 1/14
    b. 3/5
    c. 7/10
    d. 1/20

3. 3.14 + 2.73 + 23.7 =

    a. 28.57
    b. 30.57
    c. 29.56
    d. 29.57

4. A woman spent 15% of her income on an item and ends up with $120. What percentage of her income is left?

    a. 12%
    b. 85%
    c. 75%
    d. 95%

5. Express 0.27 + 0.33 as a fraction.

    a. 3/6
    b. 4/7
    c. 3/5
    d. 2/7

6. What is (3.13 + 7.87) X 5?

    a. 65
    b. 50
    c. 45
    d. 55

7. Reduce 2/4 X 3/4 to lowest terms.

    a. 6/12
    b. 3/8
    c. 6/16
    d. 3/4

8. 2/3 – 2/5 =

    a. 4/10
    b. 1/15
    c. 3/7
    d. 4/15

9. 2/7 + 2/3 =

    a. 12/23
    b. 5/10
    c. 20/21
    d. 6/21

10. 2/3 of 60 + 1/5 of 75 =

    a. 45
    b. 55
    c. 15
    d. 50

11. 8 is what percent of 40?

    a. 10%
    b. 15%
    c. 20%
    d. 25%

12. 9 is what percent of 36?

    a. 10%
    b. 15%
    c. 20%
    d. 25%

13. Three tenths of 90 equals:

    a. 18
    b. 45
    c. 27
    d. 36

14. .4% of 36 is

    a. 1.44
    b. .144
    c. 14.4
    d. 144

15. If y = 4 and x = 3, solve yx^3

   a. -108
   b. 108
   c. 27
   d. 4

16. Convert 0.007 kilograms to grams

   a. 7 grams
   b. 70 grams
   c. 0.07 grams
   d. 0.70 grams

17. Convert 16 quarts to gallons

   a. 1 gallons
   b. 8 gallons
   c. 4 gallons
   d. 4.5 gallons

18. Convert 2 teaspoons to milliliters.

   a. 4.3 milliliters
   b. 9 milliliters
   c. 9.86 milliliters
   d. 4 milliliters

19. Convert 200 meters to kilometers

   a. 50 kilometers
   b. 20 kilometers
   c. 12 kilometers
   d. 0.2 kilometers

Practice Test Questions Set 1

20. Convert 72 inches to feet
   a. 12 feet
   b. 6 feet
   c. 4 feet
   d. 17 feet

21. Convert 3 yards to feet
   a. 18 feet
   b. 12 feet
   c. 9 feet
   d. 27 feet

22. Convert 45 kg. to pounds.
   a. 10 pounds
   b. 100 pounds
   c. 1,000 pounds
   d. 110 pounds

23. Convert 0.63 grams to mg.
   a. 630 g.
   b. 63 mg.
   c. 630 mg.
   d. 603 mg.

24. 5x + 3 = 7x -1. Find x
   a. 1/3
   b. ½
   c. 1
   d. 2

25. 5x+2(x+7) = 14x − 7. Find x

   a. 1
   b. 2
   c. 3
   d. 4

26. 12t −10 = 14t + 2. Find t

   a. -6
   b. -4
   c. 4
   d. 6

27. 5(z+1) = 3(z+2) + 11. Z=?

   a. 2
   b. 4
   c. 6
   d. 12

28. The price of a book went up from $20 to $25. What percent did the price increase?

   a. 5%
   b. 10%
   c. 20%
   d. 25%

Practice Test Questions Set 1   35

29. The price of a book decreased from $25 to $20. What percent did the price decrease?

    a. 5%
    b. 10%
    c. 20%
    d. 25%

30. After taking several practice tests, Brian improved the results of his GRE test by 30%. Given that the first time he took the test Brian answered 150 questions correctly, how many questions did he answer correctly on the second test?

    a. 105
    b. 120
    c. 180
    d. 195

31. A local baseball team has 4 players (or 12.5% of the team) with long hair and the rest have short hair. How many short-haired players are there on the team?

    a. 24
    b. 28
    c. 32
    d. 50

32. In the time required to serve 43 customers, a server breaks 2 glasses and slips 5 times. The next day, the same server breaks 10 glasses. How many customers did she serve?

    a. 25
    b. 43
    c. 86
    d. 215

33. A square lawn has an area of 62,500 square meters. What will the cost of building fence around it at a rate of $5.5 per meter?

    a. $4000
    b. $4500
    c. $5000
    d. $5500

34. Mr. Brown bought 5 cheese burgers, 3 drinks, and 4 fries for his family, and a cookie pack for his dog. If the price of all single items is the same at $1.30 and a 3.5% tax is added, what is the total cost of dinner for Mr. Brown?

    a. $16
    b. $16.9
    c. $17
    d. $17.5

35. The length of a rectangle is twice of its width and its area is equal to the area of a square with 12 cm. sides. What will be the perimeter of the rectangle to the nearest whole number?

    a. 36 cm
    b. 46 cm
    c. 51 cm
    d. 56 cm

36. There are 15 yellow and 35 orange balls in a basket. How many more yellow balls must be added to make the yellow balls 65%?

    a. 35
    b. 50
    c. 65
    d. 70

37. A farmer wants to plant 65,536 trees in such a way that number of rows must be equal to the number of plants in a row. How many trees should he plant in a row?

    a. 1684

    b. 1268

    c. 668

    d. 256

38. A distributor purchased 550 kilograms of potatoes for $165. He distributed these at a rate of $6.4 per 20 kilograms to 15 shops, $3.4 per 10 kilograms to 12 shops and the remainder at $1.8. If his distribution cost is $10, what will be his profit?

    a. $10.4

    b. $24.60

    c. $14.9

    d. $23.4

39. How much pay does Mr. Johnson receive if he gives half of his pay to his family, $250 to his landlord, and has exactly 3/7 of his pay left over?

    a. $3600

    b. $3500

    c. $2800

    d. $1750

40. A boy has 4 red, 5 green and 2 yellow balls. He chooses two balls randomly. What is the probability that one is red and other is green?

    a. 2/11

    b. 19/22

    c. 20/121

    d. 9/11

Section III - English

1. Choose the sentence with the correct grammar.

a. Don would never have thought of that book, but you could have reminded him.

b. Don would never of thought of that book, but you could have reminded him.

c. Don would never have thought of that book, but you could of have reminded him.

d. Don would never of thought of that book, but you could of reminded him.

2. Choose the sentence with the correct grammar.

a. The mother would not of punished her daughter if she could have avoided it.

b. The mother would not have punished her daughter if she could of avoided it.

c. The mother would not of punished her daughter if she could of avoided it.

d. The mother would not have punished her daughter if she could have avoided it.

3. Choose the sentence with the correct grammar.

a. There was scarcely no food in the pantry, because nobody ate at home.

b. There was scarcely any food in the pantry, because nobody ate at home.

c. There was scarcely any food in the pantry, because not nobody ate at home.

d. There was scarcely no food in the pantry, because not nobody ate at home.

Practice Test Questions Set 1

4. Choose the sentence with the correct grammar.

a. Although you may not see nobody in the dark, it does not mean that nobody is there.

b. Although you may not see anyone in the dark, it does not mean that not nobody is there.

c. Although you may not see anyone in the dark, it does not mean that no one is there.

d. Although you may not see nobody in the dark, it does not mean that not nobody is there.

5. Choose the sentence with the correct grammar.

a. Michael has lived in that house for forty years, while I has owned this one for only six weeks.

b. Michael have lived in that house for forty years, while I have owned this one for only six weeks.

c. Michael have lived in that house for forty years, while I has owned this one for only six weeks.

d. Michael has lived in that house for forty years, while I have owned this one for only six weeks.

6. Choose the sentence with the correct grammar.

a. The older children have already eat their dinner, but the baby has not yet eaten anything.

b. The older children have already eaten their dinner, but the baby has not yet ate anything.

c. The older children have already eaten their dinner, but the baby has not yet eaten anything.

d. The older children have already eat their dinner, but the baby has not yet ate anything.

7. Choose the sentence with the correct grammar.

a. If they had gone to the party, he would have gone, too.

b. If they had went to the party, he would have gone, too.

c. If they had gone to the party, he would have went, too.

d. If they had went to the party, he would have went, too.

8. Choose the sentence with the correct grammar.

a. He should have went to the appointment; instead, he went to the beach.

b. He should have gone to the appointment; instead, he went to the beach.

c. He should have went to the appointment; instead, he gone to the beach.

d. He should have gone to the appointment; instead, he gone to the beach.

9. Choose the sentence with the correct grammar.

a. Lee pronounced it's name incorrectly; it's an impatiens, not an impatience.

b. Lee pronounced its name incorrectly; its an impatiens, not an impatience.

c. Lee pronounced it's name incorrectly; its an impatiens, not an impatience.

d. Lee pronounced its name incorrectly; it's an impatiens, not an impatience.

10. Choose the sentence with the correct grammar.

a. Its important for you to know its official name; its called the Confederate Museum.

b. It's important for you to know it's official name; it's called the Confederate Museum.

c. It's important for you to know its official name; it's called the Confederate Museum.

d. Its important for you to know it's official name; it's called the Confederate Museum.

11. The Ford Motor Company was named for Henry Ford, _____.

a. which had founded the company.

b. who founded the company.

c. whose had founded the company.

d. whom had founded the company.

12. Thomas Edison _____ since he invented the light bulb, television, motion pictures, and phonograph.

a. has always been known as the greatest inventor

b. was always been known as the greatest inventor

c. must have had been always known as the greatest inventor

d. will had been known as the greatest inventor

13. The weatherman on Channel 6 said that this has been the _____.

a. most hotter summer on record

b. most hottest summer on record

c. hottest summer on record

d. hotter summer on record

14. Although Joe is tall for his age, his brother Elliot is _____ of the two.

    a. the tallest
    b. more tallest
    c. the tall
    d. the taller

15. When KISS came to town, all of the tickets _____ before I could buy one.

    a. will be sold out
    b. had been sold out
    c. were being sold out
    d. was sold out

16. The rules of most sports _____ more complicated than we often realize.

    a. are
    b. is
    c. was
    d. has been

17. Neither of the Wright Brothers _____ that they would be successful with their flying machine.

    a. have any doubts
    b. has any doubts
    c. had any doubts
    d. will have any doubts

18. The Titanic _____ mere days into its maiden voyage.

    a. has already sunk
    b. will already sunk
    c. already sank
    d. sank

19. _____ won first place in the Western Division?

    a. Who
    b. Whom
    c. Which
    d. What

20. There are now several ways to listen to music, including radio, CDs, and Mp3 files _____ you can download onto an MP3 player.

    a. on which
    b. who
    c. whom
    d. which

21. As the tallest monument in the United States, the St. Louis Arch _____.

    a. has rose to an impressive 630 feet.
    b. is risen to an impressive 630 feet.
    c. rises to an impressive 630 feet.
    d. was rose to an impressive 630 feet.

22. The tired, old woman should _____ on the sofa.

    a. lie
    b. lays
    c. laid
    d. lain

23. Did the students understand that Thanksgiving always _____ on the fourth Thursday in November?

    a. fallen
    b. falling
    c. has fell
    d. falls

24. Collecting stamps, _____ and listening to short-wave radio were Rick's main hobbies.

    a. building models,
    b. to build models,
    c. having built models,
    d. build models,

25. Choose the sentence with the correct usage.

    a. The ceremony had an emotional effect on the groom, but the bride was not affected.

    b. The ceremony had an emotional affect on the groom, but the bride was not affected.

    c. The ceremony had an emotional effect on the groom, but the bride was not effected.

    d. The ceremony had an emotional affect on the groom, but the bride was not affected.

26. Choose the sentence with the correct usage.

a. Anna was taller then Luis, but then he grew four inches in three months.

b. Anna was taller then Luis, but than he grew four inches in three months.

c. Anna was taller than Luis, but than he grew four inches in three months.

d. Anna was taller than Luis, but then he grew four inches in three months.

27. Choose the sentence with the correct usage.

a. Their second home is in Boca Raton, but there not their for most of the year.

b. They're second home is in Boca Raton, but they're not there for most of the year.

c. Their second home is in Boca Raton, but they're not there for most of the year.

d. There second home is in Boca Raton, but they're not there for most of the year.

28. Choose the sentence with the correct usage.

a. They're going to graduate in June; after that, their best option will be to go there.

b. There going to graduate in June; after that, their best option will be to go there.

c. They're going to graduate in June; after that, there best option will be to go their.

d. Their going to graduate in June; after that, their best option will be to go there

29. Choose the sentence with the correct usage.

a. You're mistaken; that is not you're book.

b. Your mistaken; that is not your book.

c. You're mistaken; that is not your book.

d. Your mistaken; that is not you're book.

30. Choose the sentence with the correct usage.

a. You're classes are on the west side of campus, but you're living on the east side.

b. Your classes are on the west side of campus, but your living on the east side.

c. Your classes are on the west side of campus, but you're living on the east side.

d. You're classes are on the west side of campus, but you're living on the east side.

31. Choose the sentence below with the correct punctuation.

a. "My father said that he would be there on Sunday" Lee explained.

b. "My father said that he would be there on Sunday," Lee explained.

c. "My father said that he would be there on Sunday," Lee explained.

d. "My father said that he would be there on Sunday." Lee explained.

32. Choose the sentence below with the correct punctuation.

a. I own two dogs, a cat named Jeffrey, and Henry, the goldfish.

b. I own two dogs a cat, named Jeffrey, and Henry, the goldfish.

c. I own two dogs, a cat named Jeffrey; and Henry, the goldfish.

d. I own two dogs, a cat, named Jeffrey and Henry, the goldfish.

33. Choose the sentence below with the correct punctuation.

a. Marcus who won the debate tournament, is the best speaker that I know.

b. Marcus, who won the debate tournament, is the best speaker that I know.

c. Marcus who won the debate tournament is the best speaker that I know.

d. Marcus who won the debate tournament is the best speaker, that I know.

34. Choose the sentence below with the correct punctuation.

a. To make chicken soup you must first buy a chicken.

b. To make chicken soup you must first, buy a chicken.

c. To make chicken soup, you must first buy a chicken.

d. To make chicken soup; you must first buy a chicken.

35. Choose the sentence below with the correct punctuation.

a. To travel around the globe you have to drive 25,000 miles.

b. To travel around the globe, you have to drive 25000 miles.

c. To travel around the globe, you have to drive, 25000 miles.

d. To travel around the globe, you have to drive 25,000 miles.

36. Choose the sentence below with the correct punctuation.

a. The dog loved chasing bones, but never ate them; it was running that he enjoyed.

b. The dog loved chasing bones; but never ate them, it was running that he enjoyed.

c. The dog loved chasing bones, but never ate them, it was running that he enjoyed.

d. The dog loved chasing bones; but never ate them: it was running that he enjoyed.

37. Choose the sentence below with the correct punctuation.

a. He had not paid the rent, therefore, the landlord changed the locks.

b. He had not paid the rent; therefore, the landlord changed the locks.

c. He had not paid the rent, therefore; the landlord changed the locks.

d. He had not paid the rent therefore, the landlord changed the locks.

38. Choose the sentence below with the correct punctuation.

a. Jessica's father was in the Navy, so she attended schools in Newark, New Jersey, Key   West, Florida, San Diego, California, and Fairbanks, Alaska.

b. Jessica's father was in the Navy, so she attended schools in: Newark, New Jersey, Key West, Florida, San Diego, California, and Fairbanks, Alaska.

c. Jessica's father was in the Navy, so she attended schools in Newark, New Jersey; Key West, Florida; San Diego, California; and Fairbanks, Alaska.

d. Jessica's father was in the Navy, so she attended schools in Newark; New Jersey, Key West; Florida, San Diego, California, and Fairbanks, Alaska.

39. Identify the sentences or phrases which are written correctly.

    a. "stop! I forgot to bring my wallet," said Carl.

    b. "please wait for me," shouted Stacy.

    c. "what is your name?" asked the teacher.

    d. "I will submit my project tomorrow," said Mary.

40. Identify the sentences or phrases which are written correctly.

    a. Our family will visit china next year.

    b. The Children are happy to see Santa claus.

    c. We have relatives in Mexico.

    d. The great barrier reef in Australia can be seen in outer space.

Answer Key

Section 1 – Reading Comprehension

1. B
We can infer from this passage that sickness from an infectious disease can be easily transmitted from one person to another.

From the passage, "Infectious pathologies are also called communicable diseases or transmissible diseases, due to their potential of transmission from one person or species to another by a replicating agent (as opposed to a toxin)."

2. A
Two other names for infectious pathologies are communicable diseases and transmissible diseases.

From the passage, "Infectious pathologies are also called communicable diseases or transmissible diseases, due to their potential of transmission from one person or species to another by a replicating agent (as opposed to a toxin)."

3. C
Infectivity describes the ability of an organism to enter, survive and multiply in the host. This is taken directly from the passage, and is a definition type question.

Definition type questions can be answered quickly and easily by scanning the passage for the word you are asked to define.

"Infectivity" is an unusual word, so it is quick and easy to scan the passage looking for this word.

4. B
We know an infection is not synonymous with an infectious disease because an infection may not cause important clinical symptoms or impair host function.

5. C
We can infer from the passage that, a virus is too small to be seen with the naked eye. Clearly, if they are too small to be

seen with a microscope, then they are too small to be seen with the naked eye.

6. D
Viruses infect all types of organisms. This is taken directly from the passage, "Viruses infect all types of organisms, from animals and plants to bacteria and single-celled organisms."

7. C
The passage does not say exactly how many parts prions and viroids consist of. It does say, "Unlike prions and viroids, viruses consist of two or three parts ..." so we can infer they consist of either less than two or more than three parts.

8. B
A common virus spread by coughing and sneezing is Influenza.

9. C
The cumulus stage of a thunderstorm is the beginning of the thunderstorm.

This is taken directly from the passage, "The first stage of a thunderstorm is the cumulus, or developing stage."

10. D
The passage lists four ways that air is heated. One way is, heat created by water vapor condensing into liquid.

11. A
The sequence of events can be taken from these sentences:

As the moisture carried by the [1] air currents rises, it rapidly cools into liquid drops of water, which appear as cumulus clouds. As the water vapor condenses into liquid, it [2] releases heat, which warms the air. This in turn causes the air to become less dense than the surrounding dry air and [3] rise farther.

12. C
The purpose of this text is to explain when meteorologists consider a thunderstorm severe.

The main idea is the first sentence, "The United States National Weather Service classifies thunderstorms as severe when they reach a predetermined level." After the first sentence, the passage explains and elaborates on this idea. Everything is this passage is related to this idea, and there are no other major ideas in this passage that are central to the whole passage.

13. A
From this passage, we can infer that different areas and countries have different criteria for determining a severe storm.

From the passage we can see that most of the US has a criteria of, winds over 50 knots (58 mph or 93 km/h), and hail ¾ inch (2 cm). For the Central US, hail must be 1 inch (2.5 cm) in diameter. In Canada, winds must be 90 km/h or greater, hail 2 centimeters in diameter or greater, and rainfall more than 50 millimeters in 1 hour, or 75 millimeters in 3 hours.

Choice D is incorrect because the Canadian system is the same for hail, 2 centimeters in diameter.

14. C
With hail above the minimum size of 2.5 cm. diameter, the Central Region of the United States National Weather Service would issue a severe thunderstorm warning.

15. D
Clouds in space are made of different materials attracted by gravity. Clouds on Earth are made of water droplets or ice crystals.

Choice D is the best answer. Notice also that choice D is the most specific.

16. C
The main idea is the first sentence of the passage; a cloud is a visible mass of droplets or frozen crystals floating in the atmosphere above the surface of the Earth or other planetary body.

The main idea is very often the first sentence of the paragraph.

17. C
Nephology, which is the study of cloud physics.

18. C
This question asks about the process, and gives choices that can be confirmed or eliminated easily.

From the passage, "Dense, deep clouds reflect most light, so they appear white, at least from the top. Cloud droplets scatter light very efficiently, so the farther into a cloud light travels, the weaker it gets. This accounts for the gray or dark appearance at the base of large clouds."

We can eliminate choice A, since water droplets inside the cloud do not reflect light is false.

We can eliminate choice B, since, water droplets outside the cloud reflect light, it appears dark, is false.

Choice C is correct.

19. A
The correct order of ingredients is brown sugar, baking soda and chocolate chips.

20. B
Sturdy: strong, solid in structure or person. In context, Stir in chocolate chips by hand with a *sturdy* wooden spoon.

21. A
Disperse: to scatter in different directions or break up. In context, Stir until the chocolate chips and nuts are evenly *dispersed*.

22. B
You can stop stirring the nuts when they are evenly distributed. From the passage, "Stir until the chocolate chips and nuts are evenly dispersed."

23. A
Larvae spend most of their time in search of food and their food is leaves.

24. B
From the passage, the ants provide some degree of protection

25. C
The association is mutual so both benefit.

26. A
Navy SEALS are the maritime component of the United States Special Operations Command (USSOCOM).

27. C
Working underwater separates SEALs from other military units. This is taken directly from the passage.

28. D
SEALs also belong to the Navy and the Coast Guard.

29. A
The CIA also participated. From the passage, the raid was conducted by a "team of 40 *CIA-led* Navy SEALS."

30. C
From the passage, "The Navy SEALs were part of the Naval Special Warfare Development Group, previously called "Team 6."

Section II – Mathematics

1. A
1/3 X 3/4 = 3/12 = 1/4

2. D
75/1500 = 15/300 = 3/60 = 1/20

Practice Test Questions Set 1   55

3. D
3.14 + 2.73 = 5.87 and 5.87 + 23.7 = 29.57

4. B
Spent 15% - 100% - 15% = 85%

5. C
To convert a decimal to a fraction, take the places of decimal as your denominator, here, 2, so in 0.27, '7' is in the 100th place, so the fraction is 27/100 and 0.33 becomes 33/100.

Next estimate the answer quickly to eliminate obvious wrong choices. 27/100 is about 1/4 and 33/100 is 1/3. 1/3 is slightly larger than 1/4, and 1/4 + 1/4 is 1/2, so the answer will be slightly larger than 1/2.

Looking at the choices, Choice A can be eliminated since 3/6 = 1/2. Choice D, 2/7 is less than 1/2 and can also be eliminated. so the answer is going to be Choice B or Choice C.

Do the calculation, 0.27 + 0.33 = 0.60 and 0.60 = 60/100 = 3/5, Choice C is correct.

6. D
3.13 + 7.87 = 11 and 11 X 5 = 55

7. B
2/4 X 3/4 = 6/16, and lowest terms = 3/8

8. D
2/3-2/5 = 10-6 /15 = 4/15

9. C
2/7 + 2/3 = 6+14 /21 (21 is the common denominator) = 20/21

10. B
2/3 x 60 = 40 and 1.5 x 75 = 15, 40 + 15 = 55

11. C
This is an easy question, and shows how you can solve some

questions without doing the calculations. The question is, 8 is what percent of 40. Take easy percentages for an approximate answer and see what you get.

10% is easy to calculate because you can drop the zero, or move the decimal point. 10% of 40 = 4, and 8 = 2 X 4, so, 8 must be 2 X 10% = 20%.

Here are the calculations which confirm the quick approximation.
8/40 = X/100 = 8 * 100 / 40X = 800/40 = X = 20

12. D
This is the same type of question which illustrates another method to solve quickly without doing the calculations. The question is, 9 is what percent of 36?

Ask, what is the relationship between 9 and 36? 9 X 4 = 36 so they are related by a factor of 4. If 9 is related to 36 by a factor of 4, then what is related to 100 (to get a percent) by a factor of 4?

To visualize:

9 X 4 = 36
Z X 4 = 100

So the answer is 25. 9 has the same relation to 36 as 25 has to 100.

Here are the calculations which confirm the quick approximation.
9/36 = X/100 = 9 * 100 / 36X = 900/36 = 25

13. C
3/10 * 90 = 3 * 90/10 = 27

14. B
4/100 * 36 = .4 * 36/100 = .144

Practice Test Questions Set 1

15. B
$(4)(3)^3 = (4)(27) = 108$

16. A
1000g = 1kg., 0.007 = 1000 x 0.007 = 7g.

17. C
4 quarts = 1 gallon, 16 quarts = 16/4 = 4 gallons

18. C
1 teaspoon = 4.93 milliliters (U.S.), 2 tp = 4.93 x 2 = 9.86 ml.

19. D
1,000 meters = 1 kilometer, 200 m = 200/1,000 = 0.2 km.

20. B
12 inches = 1 ft., 72 inches = 72/12 = 6 feet

21. C
1 yard = 3 feet, 3 yards = 3 feet x 3 = 9 feet

22. B
0.45 kg = 1 pound, 1 kg. = 1/0.45 and 45 kg = 1/0.45 x 45 = 100 pounds

23. C
1 g = 1,000 mg. 0.63 g = 0.63 x 1,000 = 630 mg.

24. D
To solve for x,
5x – 7x + 3 = -1
5x – 7x = -1 -3
-2x = -4
x = -4/ -2
x = 2

25. C
To solve for x, first simplify the equation
5x + 2x + 14 = 14x – 7
7x + 14 = 4x -7
7x – 14x + 14 = -7

$7x - 14x = -7 - 14$
$-7x = -21$
$x = -21/-7$
$x = 3$

26. A
$5z + 5 = 3z + 6 + 11$
$5z - 3z + 5 = 6 + 11$
$5z - 3z = 6 + 11 - 5$
$2z = 17 - 5$
$2z = 12$
$z = 12/2$
$z = 6$

27. C
$5z + 5 = 3z + 6 + 11$
$5z - 3z + 5 = 6 + 11$
$5z - 3z = 6 + 11 - 5$
$2z = 17 - 5$
$2z = 12$
$z = 12/2$
$z = 6$

28. D
Price increased by $5 ($25-$20). The percent increase is $5/20 \times 100 = 5 \times 5 = 25\%$

29. C
Price decreased by $5 ($25-$20). The percent increase $= 5/25 \times 100 = 5 \times 4 = 20\%$

30. D
$30/100 \times 150 = 3 \times 15 = 45$ (increase in number of correct answers). So the number of correct answers in second test = $150 + 45 = 195$

31. B
Let total number of players= X
Let the number of players with long hair=Y and the number of players with short hair=Z

Then X = 4+Z
Y = 12% of X
Z = X - 4
12.5% of X = 4
Converting from decimal to fraction gives 12.5%=125/10 x 1/100=125/1000, therefore 12.5% of =125/1000X=4
Solve for X by multiplying both sides by 1000/125, X=4 x 1000/125=32
Z = x – 4
Z = 32 – 4
z or number of short haired players = 28

32. D
2 glasses are broken for 43 customers so 1 glass breaks for every 43/2 customers served, therefore 10 glasses implies 43/2 x 10=215

33. D
As the lawn is square, the length of one side will be = $\sqrt{62500}$ = 250 meters. Therefore, the perimeters will be: 250 × 4 = 1000 meters
The total cost will be 1000 × 5.5 = $5500

34. D
The price of all the single items is same and there are 13 total items. So the total cost will be 13 × 1.3 = $16.9. After 3.5 percent tax this amount will become 16.9 × 1.035 = $17.5.

35. C
Area of the square = 12 × 12 = 144 cm^2
Let x be the width, then 2x be the length of rectangle, so its area will be 2x^2 and perimeter will be 2(2x+x)=6x
According to the condition
2x^2 = 144
X = 8.48 cm
The perimeter will be
Perimeter=6×8.48
=50.88
=51 cm.

36. B
There are 50 balls in the basket now. Let x be the number of yellow balls to be added to make 65%. So the equation becomes

X + 15 /X + 50 = 65/100
X = 50

37. D
Let x be number of rows, and number of trees in a row. So equation becomes
X^2 = 65536
X = 256

38. B
First calculate the number of stores to distribute 5 kg portions: 550 - (20 x 15) - (10 x 12) = 130. Then 130/5 = 26 shops. His distribution is then: 15 x 6.4 = $96, 12 x 3.4 = $40.8, 26 x 1.8 × 26 = $46.8, Total = $183.6. Then subtract the distribution costs: Total number of stores = 15 + 12 + 26 = 53, 53 x 3 = $159 distribution costs. Then calculate profit: $183.6 - 159 = $24.60

39. B
X/2 – 250 = 3X/7
X = $3500

40. A
The probability that the 1st ball drawn is red = 4/11
The probability that the 2nd ball drawn is green = 5/10
The combined probability will then be 4/11 X 5/10 = 20/110 = 2/11

Section III English

1. A
The third conditional is used for talking about an unreal situation (a situation that did not happen) in the past. For example, "If I had studied harder, [if clause] I would have passed

the exam" [main clause]. This has the same meaning as, "I failed the exam, because I didn't study hard enough."

2. D
The third conditional is used for talking about an unreal situation (a situation that did not happen) in the past. For example, "If I had studied harder, [if clause] I would have passed the exam" [main clause]. This has the same meaning as, "I failed the exam, because I didn't study hard enough."

3. B
In double negative sentences, one of the negatives is replaced with "any."

4. C
In double negative sentences, one of the negatives is replaced with "any."

5. D
The present perfect tense cannot be used with specific time expressions such as yesterday, one year ago, last week, when I was a child, at that moment, that day, one day, etc. The present perfect tense is used with unspecific expressions such as ever, never, once, many times, several times, before, so far, already, yet, etc.

6. C
The present perfect tense cannot be used with specific time expressions such as yesterday, one year ago, last week, when I was a child, at that moment, that day, one day, etc. The present perfect tense is used with unspecific expressions such as ever, never, once, many times, several times, before, so far, already, yet, etc.

7. A
"Went" is used in the simple past tense. "Gone" is used in the past perfect tense.

8. B
"Went" is used in the simple past tense. "Gone" is used in the past perfect tense.

9. D
"It's" is a contraction for it is or it has. "Its" is a possessive pronoun.

10. C
"It's" is a contraction for it is or it has. "Its" is a possessive pronoun.

11. B
The sentence refers to a person, so "who" is the only correct choice.

12. A
The sentence requires the past perfect "has always been known." Furthermore, this is the only grammatically correct choice.

13. C
The superlative, "hottest," is used when expressing a temperature greater than that of anything to which it is being compared.

14. D
When comparing two items, use "the taller." When comparing more than two items, use "the tallest."

15. B
The past perfect form is used to describe an event that occurred in the past and prior to another event. Here there are two things that happened, both of them in the past, and something the person wanted to do.

Event 1: Kiss came to town
Event 2: All the tickets sold out
What I wanted to do: Buy a ticket

The events are arranged:

When KISS came to town, all of the tickets had been sold out before I could buy one.

16. A

The subject is "rules" so the present tense plural form, "are," is used to agree with "realize."

17. C

The simple past tense, "had," is correct because it refers to completed action in the past.

18. D

The simple past tense, "sank," is correct because it refers to completed action in the past.

19. A

"Who" is correct because the question uses an active construction. "To whom was first place given?" is passive construction.

20. D

"Which" is correct, because the files are objects and not people.

21. C

The simple present tense, "rises," is correct.

22. A

"Lie" does not require a direct object, while "lay" does. The old woman might lie on the couch, which has no direct object, or she might lay the book down, which has the direct object, "the book."

23. D

The simple present tense, "falls," is correct because it is repeated action.

24. A

The present progressive, "building models," is correct in this sentence; it is required to match the other present progressive verbs.

25. A

"Affect" is a verb, while "effect" is a noun.

26. D
"Than" is used for comparison. "Then" is used to indicate a point in time.

27. C
"There" indicates a state of existence. "Their" is used for third person plural possession. "They're" is the contracted form of "they are."

28. A
"There" indicates a state of existence. "Their" is used for third person plural possession. "They're" is the contraction of "they are."

29. C
"Your" is the possessive form of "you." "You're" is the contraction of "you are."

30. C
"Your" is the possessive form of "you." "You're" is the contraction of "you are."

31. C
Commas always go with a quote and the use of said, explained etc.

32. A
This is an example if a comma which appears before 'and,' but is disambiguating. Without the comma the sentence would be "I own two dogs, a cat named Jeffrey and Henry, the goldfish." This means there is a cat named Jeffrey and Henry, and a goldfish with no name mentioned. The comma appears to show the distinction.

I own two dogs, a cat named Jeffrey, and Henry, the goldfish.

33. B
Comma separate phrases.

34. C
Comma separate phrases.

35. B
To travel around the globe, you have to drive 25,000 miles.

36. A
The dog loved chasing bones, but never ate them; it was running that he enjoyed.

38. B
The semicolon links independent clauses with a conjunction (therefore).

39. C
The semicolon is used in a list where the list items have internal punctuation, such as "Key West, Florida."

39. D
Always capitalize the first word of a quoted sentence.

40. C
Capitalize a proper noun.

Practice Test Questions Set 2

THE PRACTICE TEST PORTION PRESENTS QUESTIONS THAT ARE REPRESENTATIVE OF THE TYPE OF QUESTION YOU SHOULD EXPECT TO FIND ON THE NET. However, they are not intended to match exactly what is on the NET.

For the best results, take this Practice Test as if it were the real exam. Set aside time when you will not be disturbed, and a location that is quiet and free of distractions. Read the instructions carefully, read each question carefully, and answer to the best of your ability.

Use the bubble answer sheets provided. When you have completed the Practice Test, check your answer against the Answer Key and read the explanation provided.

NOTE: The Reading Comprehension and English sections are optional. Check with your school for exam details.

Reading Comprehension Answer Sheet

1. Ⓐ Ⓑ Ⓒ Ⓓ 11. Ⓐ Ⓑ Ⓒ Ⓓ 21. Ⓐ Ⓑ Ⓒ Ⓓ
2. Ⓐ Ⓑ Ⓒ Ⓓ 12. Ⓐ Ⓑ Ⓒ Ⓓ 22. Ⓐ Ⓑ Ⓒ Ⓓ
3. Ⓐ Ⓑ Ⓒ Ⓓ 13. Ⓐ Ⓑ Ⓒ Ⓓ 23. Ⓐ Ⓑ Ⓒ Ⓓ
4. Ⓐ Ⓑ Ⓒ Ⓓ 14. Ⓐ Ⓑ Ⓒ Ⓓ 24. Ⓐ Ⓑ Ⓒ Ⓓ
5. Ⓐ Ⓑ Ⓒ Ⓓ 15. Ⓐ Ⓑ Ⓒ Ⓓ 25. Ⓐ Ⓑ Ⓒ Ⓓ
6. Ⓐ Ⓑ Ⓒ Ⓓ 16. Ⓐ Ⓑ Ⓒ Ⓓ 26. Ⓐ Ⓑ Ⓒ Ⓓ
7. Ⓐ Ⓑ Ⓒ Ⓓ 17. Ⓐ Ⓑ Ⓒ Ⓓ 27. Ⓐ Ⓑ Ⓒ Ⓓ
8. Ⓐ Ⓑ Ⓒ Ⓓ 18. Ⓐ Ⓑ Ⓒ Ⓓ 28. Ⓐ Ⓑ Ⓒ Ⓓ
9. Ⓐ Ⓑ Ⓒ Ⓓ 19. Ⓐ Ⓑ Ⓒ Ⓓ 29. Ⓐ Ⓑ Ⓒ Ⓓ
10. Ⓐ Ⓑ Ⓒ Ⓓ 20. Ⓐ Ⓑ Ⓒ Ⓓ 30. Ⓐ Ⓑ Ⓒ Ⓓ

Math Answer Sheet

1. A B C D   21. A B C D
2. A B C D   22. A B C D
3. A B C D   23. A B C D
4. A B C D   24. A B C D
5. A B C D   25. A B C D
6. A B C D   26. A B C D
7. A B C D   27. A B C D
8. A B C D   28. A B C D
9. A B C D   29. A B C D
10. A B C D   30. A B C D
11. A B C D   31. A B C D
12. A B C D   32. A B C D
13. A B C D   33. A B C D
14. A B C D   34. A B C D
15. A B C D   35. A B C D
16. A B C D   36. A B C D
17. A B C D   37. A B C D
18. A B C D   38. A B C D
19. A B C D   39. A B C D
20. A B C D   40. A B C D

English Grammar Answer Sheet

1. Ⓐ Ⓑ Ⓒ Ⓓ 21. Ⓐ Ⓑ Ⓒ Ⓓ
2. Ⓐ Ⓑ Ⓒ Ⓓ 22. Ⓐ Ⓑ Ⓒ Ⓓ
3. Ⓐ Ⓑ Ⓒ Ⓓ 23. Ⓐ Ⓑ Ⓒ Ⓓ
4. Ⓐ Ⓑ Ⓒ Ⓓ 24. Ⓐ Ⓑ Ⓒ Ⓓ
5. Ⓐ Ⓑ Ⓒ Ⓓ 25. Ⓐ Ⓑ Ⓒ Ⓓ
6. Ⓐ Ⓑ Ⓒ Ⓓ 26. Ⓐ Ⓑ Ⓒ Ⓓ
7. Ⓐ Ⓑ Ⓒ Ⓓ 27. Ⓐ Ⓑ Ⓒ Ⓓ
8. Ⓐ Ⓑ Ⓒ Ⓓ 28. Ⓐ Ⓑ Ⓒ Ⓓ
9. Ⓐ Ⓑ Ⓒ Ⓓ 29. Ⓐ Ⓑ Ⓒ Ⓓ
10. Ⓐ Ⓑ Ⓒ Ⓓ 30. Ⓐ Ⓑ Ⓒ Ⓓ
11. Ⓐ Ⓑ Ⓒ Ⓓ 31. Ⓐ Ⓑ Ⓒ Ⓓ
12. Ⓐ Ⓑ Ⓒ Ⓓ 32. Ⓐ Ⓑ Ⓒ Ⓓ
13. Ⓐ Ⓑ Ⓒ Ⓓ 33. Ⓐ Ⓑ Ⓒ Ⓓ
14. Ⓐ Ⓑ Ⓒ Ⓓ 34. Ⓐ Ⓑ Ⓒ Ⓓ
15. Ⓐ Ⓑ Ⓒ Ⓓ 35. Ⓐ Ⓑ Ⓒ Ⓓ
16. Ⓐ Ⓑ Ⓒ Ⓓ 36. Ⓐ Ⓑ Ⓒ Ⓓ
17. Ⓐ Ⓑ Ⓒ Ⓓ 37. Ⓐ Ⓑ Ⓒ Ⓓ
18. Ⓐ Ⓑ Ⓒ Ⓓ 38. Ⓐ Ⓑ Ⓒ Ⓓ
19. Ⓐ Ⓑ Ⓒ Ⓓ 39. Ⓐ Ⓑ Ⓒ Ⓓ
20. Ⓐ Ⓑ Ⓒ Ⓓ 40. Ⓐ Ⓑ Ⓒ Ⓓ

Section I - Reading Comprehension

Questions 1 - 4 refer to the following passage.

Passage 1 - The Respiratory System

The respiratory system's function is to allow oxygen exchange through all parts of the body. The anatomy or structure of the exchange system, and the uses of the exchanged gases, varies depending on the organism. In humans and other mammals, for example, the anatomical features of the respiratory system include airways, lungs, and the respiratory muscles. Molecules of oxygen and carbon dioxide are passively exchanged, by diffusion, between the gaseous external environment and the blood. This exchange process occurs in the alveolar region of the lungs.

Other animals, such as insects, have respiratory systems with very simple anatomical features, and in amphibians even the skin plays a vital role in gas exchange. Plants also have respiratory systems but the direction of gas exchange can be opposite to that of animals.

The respiratory system can also be divided into physiological, or functional, zones. These include the conducting zone (the region for gas transport from the outside atmosphere to just above the alveoli), the transitional zone, and the respiratory zone (the alveolar region where gas exchange occurs). [10]

1. What can we infer from the first paragraph in this passage?

 a. Human and mammal respiratory systems are the same

 b. The lungs are an important part of the respiratory system

 c. The respiratory system varies in different mammals

 d. Oxygen and carbon dioxide are passive exchanged by the respiratory system

Practice Test Questions Set 2

2. What is the process by which molecules of oxygen and carbon dioxide are passively exchanged?

    a. Transfusion
    b. Affusion
    c. Diffusion
    d. Respiratory confusion

3. What organ plays an important role in gas exchange in amphibians?

    a. The skin
    b. The lungs
    c. The gills
    d. The mouth

4. What are the three physiological zones of the respiratory system?

    a. Conducting, transitional, respiratory zones
    b. Redacting, transitional, circulatory zones
    c. Conducting, circulatory, inhibiting zones
    d. Transitional, inhibiting, conducting zones

Questions 5 - 8 refer to the following passage.

ABC Electric Warranty

ABC Electric Company warrants that its products are free from defects in material and workmanship. Subject to the conditions and limitations set forth below, ABC Electric will, at its option, either repair or replace any part of its products that prove defective due to improper workmanship or materials.

This limited warranty does not cover any damage to the

product from improper installation, accident, abuse, misuse, natural disaster, insufficient or excessive electrical supply, abnormal mechanical or environmental conditions, or any unauthorized disassembly, repair, or modification.

This limited warranty also does not apply to any product on which the original identification information has been altered, or removed, has not been handled or packaged correctly, or has been sold as second-hand.

This limited warranty covers only repair, replacement, refund or credit for defective ABC Electric products, as provided above.

5. I tried to repair my ABC Electric blender, but could not, so can I get it repaired under this warranty?

    a. Yes, the warranty still covers the blender

    b. No, the warranty does not cover the blender

    c. Uncertain. ABC Electric may or may not cover repairs under this warranty

6. My ABC Electric fan is not working. Will ABC Electric provide a new one or repair this one?

    a. ABC Electric will repair my fan

    b. ABC Electric will replace my fan

    c. ABC Electric could either replace or repair my fan can request either a replacement or a repair.

7. My stove was damaged in a flood. Does this warranty cover my stove?

    a. Yes, it is covered.

    b. No, it is not covered.

    c. It may or may not be covered.

    d. ABC Electric will decide if it is covered

8. Which of the following is an example of improper workmanship?

    a. Missing parts
    b. Defective parts
    c. Scratches on the front
    d. None of the above

Questions 9 – 12 refer to the following passage.

Passage 3 – Mythology

The main characters in myths are usually gods or supernatural heroes. As sacred stories, rulers and priests have traditionally endorsed their myths and as a result, myths have a close link with religion and politics. In the society where a myth originates, the natives believe the myth is a true account of the remote past. In fact, many societies have two categories of traditional narrative—(1) "true stories," or myths, and (2) "false stories," or fables.

Myths generally take place during a primordial age, when the world was still young, before achieving its current form. These stories explain how the world gained its current form and why the culture developed its customs, institutions, and taboos. Closely related to myth are legend and folktale. Myths, legends, and folktales are different types of traditional stories. Unlike myths, folktales can take place at any time and any place, and the natives do not usually consider them true or sacred. Legends, on the other hand, are similar to myths in that many people have traditionally considered them true. Legends take place in a more recent time, when the world was much as it is today. In addition, legends generally feature humans as their main characters, whereas myths have superhuman characters. [11]

9. We can infer from this passage that

a. Folktales took place in a time far past, before civilization covered the earth

b. Humankind uses myth to explain how the world was created

c. Myths revolve around gods or supernatural beings; the local community usually accepts these stories as not true

d. The only difference between a myth and a legend is the time setting of the story

10. The main purpose of this passage is

a. To distinguish between many types of traditional stories, and explain the back-ground of some traditional story categories

b. To determine whether myths and legends might be true accounts of history

c. To show the importance of folktales how these traditional stories made life more bearable in harder times

d. None of the Above

11. How are folktales different from myths?

a. Folktales and myth are the same

b. Folktales are not true and generally not sacred and take place anytime

c. Myths are not true and generally not sacred and take place anytime

d. Folktales explained the formation of the world and myths do not

12. How are legends and myth similar?

a. Many people believe legends and myths are true, myths take place in modern day, and legends are about ordinary people

b. Many people believe legends and myths are true, legends take place in modern day, and legends are about ordinary people

c. Many people believe legends and myths are true, legends take place in modern day, and myths are about ordinary people

d. Many people believe legends and myths are not true, legends take place in mod-ern day, and legends are about ordinary people

Questions 13 - 16 refer to the following passage.

Passage 4 – Myths, Legend and Folklore

Cultural historians draw a distinction between myth, legend and folktale simply as a way to group traditional stories. However, in many cultures, drawing a sharp line between myths and legends is not that simple. Instead of dividing their traditional stories into myths, legends, and folktales, some cultures divide them into two categories. The first category roughly corresponds to folktales, and the second is one that combines myths and legends. Similarly, we cannot always separate myths from folktales. One society might consider a story true, making it a myth. Another society may believe the story is fiction, which makes it a folktale. In fact, when a myth loses its status as part of a religious system, it often takes on traits more typical of folktales, with its formerly divine characters now appearing as human heroes, giants, or fairies. Myth, legend, and folktale are only a few of the categories of traditional stories. Other categories include anecdotes and some kinds of jokes. Traditional stories, in turn, are only one category within the much larger category of folklore, which also includes items such as gestures, costumes, and music. [11]

13. The main idea of this passage is that

  a. Myths, fables, and folktales are not the same thing, and each describes a specific type of story

  b. Traditional stories can be categorized in different ways by different people

  c. Cultures use myths for religious purposes, and when this is no longer true, the people forget and discard these myths

  d. Myths can never become folk tales, because one is true, and the other is false

14. The terms myth and legend are

  a. Categories that are synonymous with true and false

  b. Categories that group traditional stories according to certain characteristics

  c. Interchangeable, because both terms mean a story that is passed down from generation to generation

  d. Meant to distinguish between a story that involves a hero and a cultural message and a story meant only to entertain

15. Traditional story categories not only include myths and legends, but

  a. Can also include gestures, since some cultures passed these down before the written and spoken word

  b. In addition, folklore refers to stories involving fables and fairy tales

  c. These story categories can also include folk music and traditional dress

  d. Traditional stories themselves are a part of the larger category of folklore, which may also include costumes, gestures, and music

16. This passage shows that

   a. There is a distinct difference between a myth and a legend, although both are folktales

   b. Myths are folktales, but folktales are not myths

   c. Myths, legends, and folktales play an important part in tradition and the past, and are a rich and colorful part of history

   d. Most cultures consider myths to be true

Questions 17 - 19 refer to the following passage.

Passage 5 – Insects

Humans regard certain insects as pests and attempt to control them with insecticides and many other techniques. Some insects damage crops by feeding on sap, leaves or fruits, a few bite humans and livestock, alive and dead, to feed on blood and some are capable of transmitting diseases to humans, pets and live-stock. Many other insects are considered ecologically beneficial and a few provide direct economic benefit. Silkworms and bees, for example, have been domesticated for the production of silk and honey, respectively. [12]

17. How do humans control insects?

   a. By training them

   b. Using insecticides and other techniques

   c. In many different ways

   d. Humans do not control insects

18. Why do humans control insects?

   a. Because they do not like them

   b. Because they damage crops

   c. Because they damage buildings

   d. Because they damage the soil

19. How do insects damage crops?

    a. By feeding on crops

    b. By transmitting disease

    c. By laying eggs on crops

    d. None of the above

Questions 20 - 24 refer to the following passage.

Passage 6 – Trees I

Trees are an important part of the natural landscape because they prevent erosion and protect ecosystems in and under their branches. Trees also play an important role in producing oxygen and reducing carbon dioxide in the atmosphere, as well as moderating ground temperatures. Trees are important elements in landscaping and agriculture, both for their visual appeal and for their crops, such as apples, and other fruit. Wood from trees is a building material, and a primary energy source in many developing countries. Trees also play a role in many of the world's mythologies. [13]

20. What are two reasons trees are important in the natural landscape?

    a. They prevent erosion and produce oxygen

    b. They produce fruit and are important elements in landscaping

    c. Trees are not important in the natural landscape

    d. Trees produce carbon dioxide and prevent erosion

21. What kind of ecosystems do trees protect?

    a. Trees do not protect ecosystems

    b. Weather sheltered ecosystems

    c. Ecosystems around the base and under the branches

    d. All of the above

22. Which of the following is true?

a. Trees provide a primary food source in the developing world

b. Trees provide a primary building material in the developing world

c. Trees provide a primary energy source in the developing world

d. Trees provide a primary oxygen source in the developing world

23. Why are trees important for agriculture?

a. Because of their crops

b. Because they shelter ecosystems

c. Because they are a source of energy

d. Because of their visual appeal

24. What do trees do to the atmosphere?

a. Trees produce carbon dioxide and reduce oxygen

b. Trees product oxygen and carbon dioxide

c. Trees reduce oxygen and carbon dioxide

d. Trees produce oxygen and reduce carbon dioxide

Questions 25 - 28 refer to the following passage.

Passage 7 – Trees II

With an estimated 100,000 species, trees represent 25 percent of all living plant species. The majority of tree species grow in tropical regions of the world and many of these areas have not been surveyed by botanists, making species diversity poorly understood. The earliest trees were tree ferns and horsetails, which grew in forests in the Carboniferous period. Tree ferns still survive, but the only surviving horsetails are no longer in tree form. Later, in the Triassic period, conifers and ginkgos, appeared, followed by flowering plants after that in the Cretaceous period. [13]

25. Do botanists understand the number of tree species?

    a. Yes botanists know exactly how many tree species there are

    b. No, the species diversity is not well understood

    c. Yes, botanists are sure

    d. No, botanists have no idea

26. Where do most trees species grow?

    a. Most tree species grow in tropical regions.

    b. There is no one area where most tree species grow.

    c. Tree species grow in 25% of the world.

    d. There are 100,000 tree species.

27. What tree(s) survived from the Carboniferous period?

    a. 25% of all trees.

    b. Horsetails.

    c. Conifers.

    d. Tree Ferns.

28. Choose the correct list below, ranked from oldest to youngest trees.

    a. Flowering plants, conifers and ginkgos, tree ferns and horsetails.

    b. Tree ferns and horsetails, conifers and ginkgos, flowering plants.

    c. Tree ferns and horsetails, flowering plants, conifers and ginkgos.

    d. Conifers and ginkgos, tree ferns and horsetails, flowering plants.

Questions 29 - 30 refer to the following passage.

Lowest Price Guarantee

Get it for less. Guaranteed!

ABC Electric will beat any advertised price by 10% of the difference.

> 1) If you find a lower advertised price, we will beat it by 10% of the difference.
>
> 2) If you find a lower advertised price within 30 days* of your purchase we will beat it by 10% of the difference.
>
> 3) If our own price is reduced within 30 days* of your purchase, bring in your receipt and we will refund the difference.

*14 days for computers, monitors, printers, laptops, tablets, cellular & wireless devices, home security products, projectors, camcorders, digital cameras, radar detectors, portable DVD players, DJ and pro-audio equipment, and air conditioners.

29. I bought a radar detector 15 days ago and saw an ad for the same model only cheaper. Can I get 10% of the difference refunded?

> a. Yes. Since it is less than 30 days, you can get 10% of the difference refunded.
>
> b. No. Since it is more than 14 days, you cannot get 10% of the difference re-funded.
>
> c. It depends on the cashier.
>
> d. Yes. You can get the difference refunded.

30. I bought a flat-screen TV for $500 10 days ago and found an advertisement for the same TV, at another store, on sale for $400. How much will ABC refund under this guarantee?

   a. $100
   b. $110
   c. $10
   d. $400

Section II – Math

1. 8327 – 1278 =

   a. 7149
   b. 7209
   c. 6059
   d. 7049

2. 294 X 21 =

   a. 6017
   b. 6174
   c. 6728
   d. 5679

3. 1278 + 4920 =

   a. 6298
   b. 6108
   c. 6198
   d. 6098

4. 285 * 12 =

    a. 3420
    b. 3402
    c. 3024
    d. 2322

5. 4120 – 3216 =

    a. 903
    b. 804
    c. 904
    d. 1904

6. 2417 + 1004 =

    a. 3401
    b. 4321
    c. 3402
    d. 3421

7. 1440 ÷ 12 =

    a. 122
    b. 120
    c. 110
    d. 132

8. 2713 – 1308 =

    a. 1450
    b. 1445
    c. 1405
    d. 1455

9. It is known that $x^2 + 4x = 5$. Then x can be

   a. 0
   b. -5
   c. 1
   d. Either (b) or (c)

10. $(a+b)2 = 4ab$. What is necessarily correct?

   a. a > b
   b. a < b
   c. a = b
   d. None of the Above

11. The sum of the digits of a 2-digit number is 12. If we switch the digits, the number we get will be greater than the initial one by 36. Find the initial number.

   a. 39
   b. 48
   c. 57
   d. 75

12. Two friends traveled to a nearby city. In the second day they travelled 75 miles more than the first day, and in the third day, they travelled a third of the distance covered in the second day. How many miles did they cover in the first day, if the total travelled was 170 miles?

   a. 30 miles
   b. 35 miles
   c. 105 miles
   d. 135 miles

13. Kate's father is 32 years older than Kate is. In 5 years, he will be five times older. How old is Kate?

    a. 2
    b. 3
    c. 5
    d. 6

14. If Lynn can type a page in p minutes, what portion of the page can she do in 5 minutes?

    a. $5/p$
    b. $p - 5$
    c. $p + 5$
    d. $p/5$

15. If Sally can paint a house in 4 hours, and John can paint the same house in 6 hours, how long will it take for both of them to paint the house together?

    a. 2 hours and 24 minutes
    b. 3 hours and 12 minutes
    c. 3 hours and 44 minutes
    d. 4 hours and 10 minutes

16. Employees of a discount appliance store receive an additional 20% off the lowest price on any item. If an employee purchases a dishwasher during a 15% off sale, how much will he pay if the dishwasher originally cost $450?

    a. $280.90
    b. $287
    c. $292.50
    d. $306

17. The sale price of a car is $12,590, which is 20% off the original price. What is the original price?

    a. $14,310.40
    b. $14,990.90
    c. $15,108.00
    d. $15,737.50

18. A goat eats 214 kg. of hay in 60 days, while a cow eats the same amount in 15 days. How long will it take them to eat this hay together?

    a. 37.5
    b. 75
    c. 12
    d. 15

19. Express 25% as a fraction.

    a. 1/4
    b. 7/40
    c. 6/25
    d. 8/28

20. Express 125% as a decimal.

    a. .125
    b. 12.5
    c. 1.25
    d. 125

21. Solve for x: 30 is 40% of x

    a. 60
    b. 90
    c. 85
    d. 75

Practice Test Questions Set 2

22. 12 ½% of x is equal to 50. Solve for x.

   a. 300
   b. 400
   c. 450
   d. 350

23. Express 24/56 as a reduced common fraction.

   a. 4/9
   b. 4/11
   c. 3/7
   d. 3/8

24. Express 87% as a decimal.

   a. .087
   b. 8.7
   c. .87
   d. 87

25. 60 is 75% of x. Solve for x.

   a. 80
   b. 90
   c. 75
   d. 70

26. 60% of x is 12. Solve for x.

   a. 18
   b. 15
   c. 25
   d. 20

27. Express 71/1000 as a decimal.

   a. .71
   b. .0071
   c. .071
   d. 7.1

28. 4.7 + .9 + .01 =

   a. 5.5
   b. 6.51
   c. 5.61
   d. 5.7

29. .33 × .59 =

   a. .1947
   b. 1.947
   c. .0197
   d. .1817

30. .84 ÷ .7 =

   a. .12
   b. 12
   c. .012
   d. 1.2

31. What number is in the ten thousandths place in 1.7389?

   a. 1
   b. 8
   c. 9
   d. 3

32. .87 - .48 =

   a. .39
   b. .49
   c. .41
   d. .37

33. The manager of a weaving factory estimates that if 10 machines run on 100% efficiency for 8 hours, they will produce 1450 meters of cloth. However, due to some technical problems, 4 machines run of 95% efficiency and the remaining 6 at 90% efficiency. How many meters of cloth can these machines will produce in 8 hours?

   a. 1479 meters
   b. 1310 meters
   c. 1300 meters
   d. 1285 meters

34. Convert 60 feet to inches.

   a. 700 inches
   b. 600 inches
   c. 720 inches
   d. 1,800 inches

35. Convert 25 centimeters to millimeters.

   a. 250 millimeters
   b. 7.5 millimeters
   c. 5 millimeters
   d. 2.5 millimeters

36. Convert 100 millimeters to centimeters.

   a. 10 centimeters
   b. 1,000 centimeters
   c. 1100 centimeters
   d. 50 centimeters

37. Convert 3 gallons to quarts.

   a. 15 quarts
   b. 6 quarts
   c. 12 quarts
   d. 32 quarts

38. 2000 mm. =

   a. 2 m
   b. 200 m
   c. 0.002 m
   d. 0.02 m

39. 0.05 ml. =

   a. 50 liters
   b. 0.00005 liters
   c. 5 liters
   d. 0.0005 liters

40. 30 mg is the same mass as:

   a. 0.0003 kg.
   b. 0.03 grams
   c. 300 decigrams
   d. 0.3 grams

Section III – English Grammar

1. Elaine promised to bring the camera _____ at the mall yesterday.

    a. by me
    b. with me
    c. at me
    d. to me

2. Last night, he _____ the sleeping bag down beside my mattress.

    a. lay
    b. laid
    c. lain
    d. has laid

3. I would have bought the shirt for you if _____.

    a. I had known you liked it.
    b. I have known you liked it.
    c. I would know you liked it.
    d. I know you liked it.

4. Many believers still hope _____ proof of the existence of ghosts.

    a. two find
    b. to find
    c. to found
    d. to have been found

Select the correct word or phrase for the blank.

5. All the people at the school, including the teachers and _____ were glad when summer break came.

    a. students:

    b. students,

    c. students;

    d. students

6. To _____, Anne was on time for her math class.

    a. everybody's surprise

    b. every body's surprise

    c. everybodys surprise

    d. everybodys' surprise

7. If he _____ the textbook like he was supposed to, he would have known what was on the test.

    a. will have read

    b. shouldn't have read

    c. would have read

    d. had read

8. Following the tornado, telephone poles _____ all over the street.

    a. laid

    b. lied

    c. were lying

    d. were laying

Practice Test Questions Set 2

9. In Edgar Allen Poe's _____ Edgar Allen Poe describes a man with a guilty conscience.

    a. short story, "The Tell-Tale Heart,"

    b. short story The Tell-Tale Heart,

    c. short story, The Tell-Tale Heart

    d. short story. "the Tell-Tale Heart,"

10. Billboards are considered an important part of advertising for big business, _____ by their critics.

    a. but, an eyesore;

    b. but, " an eyesore,"

    c. but an eyesore

    d. but-an eyesore-

11. I can never remember how to use those two common words, "sell," meaning to trade a product for money, or _____ meaning an event where products are traded for less money than usual.

    a. sale-

    b. "sale,"

    c. "sale

    d. "to sale,"

12. The class just finished reading _____ a short story by Carl Stephenson about a plantation owner's battle with army ants.

    a. a)-"Leinengen versus the Ants,"

    b. b) Leinengen versus the Ants,

    c. c) "Leinengen versus the Ants,"

    d. c) Leinengen versus the Ants

13. After the car was fixed, it _____ again.

    a. ran good
    b. ran well
    c. would have run well
    d. ran more well

14. "Where does the sun go during the _____ asked little Kathy.

    a. night,"
    b. night"?,
    c. night,?"
    d. night?"

15. When I was a child, my mother taught me to say thank you, holding the door open for other, and cover my mouth when yawning or coughing.

    a. When I was a child, my mother teaching me to say thank you, to hold the door open for others, and cover my mouth when yawning or coughing.

    b. When I was a child, my mother taught me say thank you, to hold the door open for others, and to covering my mouth when yawning or coughing.

    c. When I was a child, my mother taught me saying thank you, holding the door open for others, and to cover my mouth when yawning or coughing.

    d. When I was a child, my mother taught me to say thank you, hold the door open for others, and cover my mouth when yawning or coughing.

16. Mother is talking to a man that wants to hire her to be a receptionist.

  a. Mother is talking to a man who wants to hire her to be a receptionist.

  b. Mother is talked to a man who wants to hire her to be a receptionist.

  c. Mother is talking to a man who wants to her. To be a receptionist.

  d. Mother is talking to a man hiring her who to be a receptionist.

17. Those comic books, which was for sale at the magazine shop, are now quite valuable.

  a. Those comics books which were for sale, at the magazine shop are now quite valuable.

  b. Those comic books, which were for sale at the magazine, shop, are now quite valuable.

  c. Those comic books, which were for sale at the magazine shop, are now, quite valuable

  d. Those comic books, which were for sale at the magazine shop, are now quite valuable.

18. If you want to sell your car, it's important being honest with the buyer.

  a. If you want to sell your car, being honest with the buyer is important.

  b. If you want to sell your car, to be honest with the buyer is important.

  c. If you wanting to sell your car, being honest with the buyer are important.

  d. If you want to selling your car, to be honest with the buyer is important.

19. Although today the boy was nice to my brother, they usually was quite mean to him.

    a. Although today the boy was nice to my brother, they were usually quite mean to him.

    b. Although today the boy was nice to my brother, he was usually quite mean to him.

    c. Although today the boy were nice to my brother, he is usually quite mean to him.

    d. Although today the boy was nice to my brother, he were usually quite mean to him.

Combine The Separate Sentences Into One Simpler Sentence With The Same Meaning.

20. The customers were impatient for the store to open. The customers rushed inside when the doors were open.

    a. Although the customers were impatient for the store to open, the doors were opened when the customers rushed inside.

    b. Although the doors were opened before customers rushed inside, the customers were impatient for the store to open.

    c. The customers, who were impatient for the store to open, rushed inside as soon as the doors were open.

    d. Although the doors were opened by impatient customers, they rushed inside before the store was open.

21. I should enter my dog in a dog pageant. Everyone says that my dog, whose name is Skipper, is the most beautiful one they've ever seen."

a. Because my dog's name is Skipper, my dog was entered in the pageant and everyone said he was the mot beautiful dog that they've ever seen.

b. I should enter my dog in a dog pageant, since everyone says that Skipper is the most beautiful dog they've ever seen.

c. Before I entered my dog in the dog pageant, Skipper said that he was the most beautiful dog that he'd ever seen.

d. Skipper entered my dog in the dog pageant because he was the most beautiful one that anyone had ever seen.

22. The doctor was not looking forward to meeting Mrs. Lucas. The doctor would have to tell Mrs. Lucas that she has cancer. The doctor hated giving bad news to patients.

a. The doctor hated giving bad news, and so he was not looking forward to meeting Mrs. Lucas because he would have to tell her that she has cancer.

b. The doctor has cancer and was not looking forward to meeting Mrs. Lucas and telling her this bad news.

c. Before the doctor met Mrs. Lucas, he had to give his the patients the bad news that Mrs. Lucas has cancer.

d. The doctor was not looking forward to giving the bad news to his patients that he had to tell Mrs. Lucas that his patients have cancer.

23. Mom hates shopping. We were out of bread, milk and eggs. Mom went to the supermarket.

a. Because we were out of bread, milk and eggs, Mom hated shopping at the supermarket.

b. Although she hates shopping, Mom went to the supermarket since we were out of bread, milk and eggs.

c. Although we were out of bread, milk and eggs, Mom still hated shopping at the supermarket and went there anyway.

d. Because Mom hated shopping at the supermarket, she went to there to buy her bread, milk and eggs.

24. I hate needles. I want to give blood. I can't give blood.

a. Although I hate needles, I can't give blood even even if I wanted to.

b. Because I hate needles, I can't give blood, although I want to.

c. Whenever I hate needles, I give blood although I can't give blood.

d. Whenever I can't give blood, I give blood anyway, although I hate needles.

25. Choose the sentence below with the correct punctuation.

a. George wrecked John's car that was the end of their friendship.

b. George wrecked John's car. that was the end of their friendship.

c. George wrecked John's car; that was the end of their friendship.

d. None of the above

26. Choose the sentence below with the correct punctuation.

a. The dress was not Gina's favorite; however, she wore it to the dance.

b. The dress was not Gina's favorite, however, she wore it to the dance.

c. The dress was not Gina's favorite, however; she wore it to the dance.

d. The dress was not Gina's favorite however, she wore it to the dance.

27. Choose the sentence below with the correct punctuation.

a. Chris showed his dedication to golf in many ways, for example, he watched all of the tournaments on television.

b. Chris showed his dedication to golf in many ways; for example, he watched all of the   tournaments on television.

c. Chris showed his dedication to golf in many ways, for example; he watched all of the tournaments on television.

d. Chris showed his dedication to golf in many ways for example he watched all of the tournaments on television.

28. Choose the sentence below with the correct punctuation.

a. There are many species of owls, the Great-Horned Owl, the Snowy Owl, and the Western Screech Owl, and the Barn Owl.

b. There are many species of owls, the Great-Horned Owl: the Snowy Owl: and the Western Screech Owl, and the Barn Owl.

c. There are many species of owls; the Great-Horned Owl, the Snowy Owl, and the Western Screech Owl, and the Barn Owl.

d. There are many species of owls: the Great-Horned Owl, the Snowy Owl, and the Western Screech Owl, and the Barn Owl.

29. Choose the sentence below with the correct punctuation.

a. In his most famous speech, Reverend King proclaimed: "I have a dream!"

b. In his most famous speech, Reverend King proclaimed; "I have a dream!"

c. In his most famous speech, Reverend King proclaimed. "I have a dream!"

d. In his most famous speech: Reverend King proclaimed, "I have a dream!"

30. Choose the sentence below with the correct punctuation.

    a. Puzzled — Joe said, "You aren't going to pay me until ?"

    b. Puzzled, Joe said, "You aren't going to pay me until ?"

    c. Puzzled, Joe said, "You aren't going to pay me until —?"

    d. Puzzled, Joe said, "You aren't going to pay me until, ?"

31. Choose the sentence below with the correct punctuation.

    a. The years of his employment were not consecutive, being from 1999 to 2001 and 2002 – 2004.

    b. The years of his employment were not consecutive, being from 1999 – 2001 and 2002 – 2004.

    c. The years of his employment were not consecutive, being from 1999 _ 2001 and 2002_ 2004.

    d. The years of his employment were not consecutive, being from 1999, 2001 and 2002, 2004.

32. Who do you think will win the contest _____

    a. .

    b. !

    c. ?

    d. ,

33. Four extra guests are coming to dinner _____

    a. .

    b. ?

    c. !

    d. ;

34. This is absolutely incredible _____

    a. !
    b. .
    c. :
    d. ;

35. Watch out for the broken glass _____

    a. .
    b. ?
    c. ,
    d. !

36. Choose the sentence with the correct usage.

    a. The ceremony had an emotional effect on the groom, but the bride was not affected.

    b. The ceremony had an emotional affect on the groom, but the bride was not affected.

    c. The ceremony had an emotional effect on the groom, but the bride was not effected.

    d. The ceremony had an emotional affect on the groom, but the bride was not affected.

37. Choose the sentence with the correct usage.

    a. Anna was taller then Luis, but then he grew four inches in three months.

    b. Anna was taller then Luis, but than he grew four inches in three months.

    c. Anna was taller than Luis, but than he grew four inches in three months.

    d. Anna was taller than Luis, but then he grew four inches in three months.

38. Choose the sentence with the correct usage.

a. Their second home is in Boca Raton, but there not their for most of the year.

b. They're second home is in Boca Raton, but they're not there for most of the year.

c. Their second home is in Boca Raton, but they're not there for most of the year.

d. There second home is in Boca Raton, but they're not there for most of the year.

39. Choose the sentence with the correct usage.

a. They're going to graduate in June; after that, their best option will be to go there.

b. There going to graduate in June; after that, their best option will be to go there.

c. They're going to graduate in June; after that, there best option will be to go their.

d. Their going to graduate in June; after that, their best option will be to go there.

40. Choose the sentence with the correct usage.

a. You're mistaken; that is not you're book.

b. Your mistaken; that is not your book.

c. You're mistaken; that is not your book.

d. Your mistaken; that is not you're book.

Answer Key

1. B
We can infer an important part of the respiratory system are the lungs. From the passage, "Molecules of oxygen and carbon dioxide are passively exchanged, by diffusion, between the gaseous external environment and the blood. This exchange process occurs in the alveolar region of the lungs."

Therefore, one of the primary functions for the respiratory system is the exchange of oxygen and carbon dioxide, and this process occurs in the lungs. We can therefore infer that the lungs are an important part of the respiratory system.

2. C
The process by which molecules of oxygen and carbon dioxide are passively exchanged is diffusion.

This is a definition type question. Scan the passage for references to "oxygen," "carbon dioxide," or "exchanged."

3. A
The organ that plays an important role in gas exchange in amphibians is the skin.

Scan the passage for references to "amphibians," and find the answer.

4. A
The three physiological zones of the respiratory system are Conducting, transitional, respiratory zones.

5. B
This warranty does not cover a product that you have tried to fix yourself. From paragraph two, "This limited warranty does not cover ... any unauthorized disassembly, repair, or modification. "

6. C
ABC Electric could either replace or repair the fan, provided the other conditions are met. ABC Electric has the option to repair or replace.

7. B
The warranty does not cover a stove damaged in a flood. From the passage, "This limited warranty does not cover any damage to the product from improper installation, accident, abuse, misuse, natural disaster, insufficient or excessive electrical supply, abnormal mechanical or environmental conditions."

A flood is an "abnormal environmental condition," and a natural disaster, so it is not covered.

8. A
A missing part is an example of defective workmanship. This is an error made in the manufacturing process. A defective part is not considered workmanship.

9. B
The first paragraph tells us that myths are a true account of the remote past.

The second paragraph tells us that, "myths generally take place during a primordial age, when the world was still young, prior to achieving its current form."

Putting these two together, we can infer that humankind used myth to explain how the world was created.

10. A
This passage is about different types of stories. First, the passage explains myths, and then compares other types of stories to myths.

11. B
From the passage, "Unlike myths, folktales can take place at any time and any place, and the natives do not usually consider them true or sacred."

12. B
This question gives options with choices for the three different characteristics of myth and legend. The options are,

- True or not true
- Takes place in modern day
- About ordinary people

For this type of question, where two things are compared for different characteristics, you can easily eliminate wrong answers using only one of the choices. Take myths: myths are believed to be true, do not take place in modern day, and are not about ordinary people.

Make a list as follows,

True or not true - True

Takes place in modern day - No

About ordinary people - No

Now check the options quickly. Option A is wrong (myths do not take place in modern day). Option B looks good. Put a check beside it. Option C is incorrect (myths are about ordinary people), and Option D is incorrect (myths are not true), so the answer must be Option B.

13. B
This passage describes the different categories for traditional stories. The other options are facts from the passage, not the main idea of the passage. The main idea of a passage will always be the most general statement. For example, Option A, Myths, fables, and folktales are not the same thing, and each describes a specific type of story. This is a true statement from the passage, but not the main idea of the passage, since the passage also talks about how some cultures may classify a story as a myth and others as a folktale.

The statement, from Option B, Traditional stories can be categorized in different ways by different people, is a more general statement that describes the passage.

14. B
Option B is the best choice, categories that group traditional

stories according to certain characteristics.

Choices A and C are false and can be eliminated right away. Choice D is designed to confuse. Choice D may be true, but it is not mentioned in the passage.

15. D
The best answer is D, traditional stories themselves are a part of the larger category of folklore, which may also include costumes, gestures, and music.

All the other choices are false. Traditional stories are part of the larger category of Folklore, which includes other things, not the other way around.

16. A
There is a distinct difference between a myth and a legend, although both are folktales.

17. B
The techniques for controlling insects are taken directly from the first sentence.

18. B
The inference is humans control pests because they damage crops.

19. A
Feeding on crops is the best choice, even though choices A and C are also correct.

20. A
Choice A is a re-wording of text from the passage.

21. B
This is taken directly from the passage.

22. C
Although trees are used as a building material, this is not their primary use. Trees are a primary energy source.

23. A
This is taken directly from the passage.

24. D
This question is designed to confuse by presenting different choices for the two chemicals, oxygen and carbon dioxide. One is produced, and one is reduced. Read the passage carefully to see which is reduced and which is produced.

25. B
The inference is botanists have not surveyed all of the tropical areas so they do not know the number of species.

26. A
This is taken directly from the passage.

27. D
Tree-ferns survived the Carboniferous period. This is a fact-based question about the Carboniferous period. "Carboniferous" is an unusual word, so the fastest way to answer this question is to scan the pas-sage for the word "Carboniferous" and find the answer.

28. B
Here is the passage with the oldest to youngest trees.

The earliest trees were [1] tree ferns and horsetails, which grew in forests in the Carboniferous period. Tree ferns still survive, but the only surviving horsetails are no longer in tree form. Later, in the Triassic period, [2] conifers and ginkgos, appeared, [3] followed by flowering plants after that in the Cretaceous period.

29. B
The time limit for radar detectors is 14 days. Since you made the purchase 15 days ago, you do not qualify for the guarantee.

Section II – Mathematics

1. D
8327 − 1278 = 7049

Practice Test Questions Set 2

2. B
294 X 21 = 6174

3. C
1278 + 4920 = 6198

4. A
285 * 12 = 3420

5. C
4120 − 3216 = 904

6. D
2417 + 1004 = 3421

7. B
1440 ÷ 12 = 120

8. C
2713 − 1308 = 1405

9. D
$x^2 + 4x = 5$, $x^2 + 4x - 5 = 0$, $x^2 + 5x - x - 5 = 0$, factorize $x(x+5) - 1(x+5) = 0$, $(x+5)(x-1)=0$. $x + 5 = 0$ or $x - 1 = 0$, $x = 0 - 5$ or $x = 0 + 1$, $x = -5$ or $x = 1$, either b or c.

10. C
Open parenthesis: 2a + 2b = 4ab, divide both sides by 2 = a+b=2ab or a+b=ab + ab, therefore a=ab and b=ab, therefore a=b.

11. B
Let the XY represent the initial number, X + Y = 12, YX=XY+ 36, Only b = 48 satisfies both equations above from the given choices.

12. A

13. B
Let the father's age = Y, and Kate's age = X, therefore Y = 32 +

X, in 5 years, y = 5x, substituting for Y will be 5x = 32 + X, 5X − X = 32, 4X = 32, X = 32/8, x = 8, Kate will be 8 in 5 years time, so Kate's present age = 8 - 5 = 3.

14. D

15. A
Let X represent the house, Sally paints X in 4 hours or ¼ X per 1hr or 60 minutes, John paints X in 6 hours or at 1/6X per 1hr or 60mins. Working together, they will paint 1/4x + 1/6x in 1hr or 60minutes = 10/24x = 5/12x every 60 minutes, to paint x = 60 minutes x 12/5 = 144 minutes or 2 hrs and 24 minutes.

16. D
The cost of the dishwasher = $450, 15% discount = 15/100 x 450 = $67.5,
The new price = 450 − 67.5 = $382.5, 20% discount on lowest price = 20/100 x 382.5 = $76.5,
so the final price = $306.

17. D
Original price = x,
80/100 = 12590/X,
80X = 1259000,
X = 15737.50.

18. C
Total hay = 214 kg,
The goat eats at a rate of 214/60 days = 3.6 kg per day.
The Cow eats at a rate of 214/15 = 14.3 kg per day,
Together they eat 3.6 + 14.3 = 17.9 per day.
At a rate of 17.9 kg per day, they will consume 214 kg in 214/17.9 = 11.96 or 12 days approx.

19. A
25% = 25/100 = 1/4

20. C
125/100 = 1.25

Practice Test Questions Set 2   111

21. D
40/100 = 30/X = 40X = 30*100 = 3000/40 = 75

22. B
12.5/100 = 50/X = 12.5X = 50 * 100 = 5000/12.5 = 400

23. C
24/56 = 3/7 (divide numerator and denominator by 8)

24. C
Converting percent to decimal – divide percent by 100 and remove the % sign. 87% = 87/100 = .87

25. A
60 has the same relation to X as 75 to 100 – so
60/X = 75/100
6000 = 75X
X = 80

26. D
60 has the same relationship to 100 as 12 does to X – so
60/100 = 12/X
1200 = 60X
X = 20

27. C
Converting a fraction into a decimal – divide the numerator by the denominator – so 71/1000 = .071. Dividing by 1000 moves the decimal point 3 places.

28. C
4.7 + .9 + .01 = 5.61

29. A
.33 × .59 = .1947

30. D
.84 ÷ .7 = 1.2

31. C
9 is in the ten thousandths place in 1.7389.

32. A
.87 - .48 = .39

33. A
At 100% efficiency 1 machine produces 1450/10 = 145 m of cloth.
At 95% efficiency, 4 machines produce 4 X 0.95 X 145 = 551 m of cloth.
At 90% efficiency, 6 machines produce 6 X 0.90 X 145 = 783 m of cloth.

Total cloth produced = 145 + 551 + 783 = 1479 m

34. C
1 foot = 12 inches, 60 feet = 60 x 12 = 720 inches.

35. A
1 centimeter = 10 millimeter, 25 centimeter = 25 X 10 = 250.

36. A
1 millimeter = 10 centimeter, 100 millimeter = 100/10 = 10 centimeters.

37. C
1 gallon = 4 quarts, 3 gallons = 3 x 4 = 12 quarts.

38. A
There are 1000 mm in a meter.

39. B
There are 1000 ml in a liter. 0.05/1000 = 0.00005 liters.

40. D
There are 1000 mg in a gram. 30/1000 = 0.03 grams.

Section IV – English Grammar

1. D
The preposition "to" is correct. "To" here means give.

2. A
"Lie" means to recline, and does not take an object. "lay" means to place and does take an object.

3. A
Past unreal conditional. Takes the form,
[If ... Past Perfect ..., ... would have + past participle ...]

4. B
This sentence is in the present tense, so "to find" is correct.

5. B
The comma separates a phrase.

6. A
Possessive pronouns ending in s take an apostrophe before the 's': one's; everyone's; somebody's, nobody else's, etc.

7. D
When talking about something that didn't happen in the past, use the past perfect (if I had done).

8. C
"Lie" means to recline, and does not take an object. "Lay" means to place and does take an object. Peter lay the books on the table (the books are the direct object), or the telephone poles were lying on the road (no direct object).

9. A
Titles of short stories are enclosed in quotation marks.

10. C
No additional punctuation is required here.

11. B
Here the word "sale" is used as a "word" and not as a word in the sentence, so quotation marks are used.

12. C
Titles of short stories are enclosed in quotation marks, and commas always go inside quotation marks.

13. B
"Ran well" is correct. "Ran good" is never correct.

14. D
Commas and periods always go inside quotation marks. Question marks that are part of a quote also go inside quotation marks; however, if the writer quotes a statement as part of a larger question, the question mark is placed after the quotation mark.

15. D
The sentence starts with a phrase, which is separated by a comma and then lists the things the speaker's mother taught, to say thank you, etc. Each of the items in the list are separated by a comma.

16. A
When referring to a person, use "who" instead of "that."

17. A
The comma separates a phrase starting with 'which.'

18. A
"Being honest," present tense is the best choice. "The buyer" is singular so use "is."

19. C
The subject in the first phrase, "the boy," has to agree with the subject in the second phrase, "he is."

20. C
These two sentences can be combined into one sentence with 2 clauses separated by a comma.

21. B
These two sentences can be combined and the phrase, 'whose name is Skipper,' deleted.

22. A
These three sentences can be combined using 'although,' and 'even if.'

23. B
These two sentences can be combined into one sentence with two clauses separated by a comma.

24. A
These three sentences can be combined using 'although,' and 'since.'

25. C
The semicolon links independent clauses.

26. A
The semicolon links independent clauses with a conjunction (However).

27. B
The semicolon links independent clauses.

28. D
A colon informs the reader that what follows the mark proves, explains, or lists elements of what preceded the mark.

29. A
A colon informs the reader that what follows the mark proves, explains, or lists elements of what preceded the mark.

30. C
The dash is used when the speaker cannot continue.

31. B
The dash is used to indicate a closed range of values.

32. C
A question mark is used to end an interrogative sentence, that is, at the end of a direct question which requires an answer.

33. B
Use a question mark to end a statement that is intended as a question.

34. A
Use an exclamation mark to end an exclamatory sentence, that is, at the end of a statement showing strong emotion.

35. D
Use an exclamation mark after an imperative sentence if the command is urgent and forceful.

36. A
"Affect" is a verb, while "effect" is a noun.

37. D
"Than" is used for comparison. "Then" is used to indicate a point in time.

38. C
"There" indicates a state of existence. "Their" is used for third person plural possession. "They're" is the contracted form of "they are."

39. A
"There" indicates a state of existence. "Their" is used for third person plural possession. "They're" is the contraction of "they are."

40. C
"Your" is the possessive form of "you." "You're" is the contraction of "you are."

Conclusion

CONGRATULATIONS! You have made it this far because you have applied yourself diligently to practicing for the exam and no doubt improved your potential score considerably! Getting into a good school is a huge step in a journey that might be challenging at times but will be many times more rewarding and fulfilling. That is why being prepared is so important.

Study then Practice and then Succeed!

Good Luck!

Thanks!

If you enjoyed this book and would like to order additional copies for yourself or for friends, please check with your local bookstore, favourite online bookseller or visit www.test-preparation.ca and place your order directly with the publisher.

Feedback to the publisher may be sent by email to feedback@test-preparation.ca

NOTES

Text where noted below is used under the Creative Commons Attribution-ShareAlike 3.0 License

http://en.wikipedia.org/wiki/Wikipedia:Text_of_Creative_Commons_Attribution-ShareAlike_3.0_Unported_License

[1] Infectious Disease. In *Wikipedia*. Retrieved November 12, 2010 from en.wikipedia.org/wiki/Infectious_disease.
[2] Virus. In *Wikipedia*. Retrieved November 12, 2010 from en.wikipedia.org/wiki/Virus.
[3] Cloud. In *Wikipedia*. Retrieved November 12, 2010 from en.wikipedia.org/wiki/Cloud.
[4] Thunderstorm. In *Wikipedia*. Retrieved November 12, 2010 from en.wikipedia.org/wiki/Thunderstorm.
[5] Butterfly. In *Wikipedia*. Retrieved November 12, 2010 from en.wikipedia.org/wiki/Butterfly.
[6] U.S. Navy Seal. In *Wikipedia*. Retrieved November 12, 2010 from en.wikipedia.org/wiki/United_States_Navy_SEALs.
[7] Respiratory System. In *Wikipedia*. Retrieved November 12, 2010 from en.wikipedia.org/wiki/Respiratory_system.
[8] Mythology. In *Wikipedia*. Retrieved November 12, 2010 from en.wikipedia.org/wiki/Mythology.
[9] Insect. In *Wikipedia*. Retrieved November 12, 2010 from en.wikipedia.org/wiki/Insect.
[10] Tree. In *Wikipedia*. Retrieved November 12, 2010 from en.wikipedia.org/wiki/Tree.

www.ingramcontent.com/pod-product-compliance
Lightning Source LLC
Chambersburg PA
CBHW061513180526
45171CB00001B/154